HAPPINESS IN MARRIAGE

HAPPINESS IN MARRIAGE

BY

MARGARET SANGER

APPLEWOOD BOOKS
Distributed by The Globe Pequot Press

Happiness in Marriage was originally published in 1926.

ISBN 1-55709-204-4

Thank you for purchasing an Applewood Book.
Applewood reprints America's lively classics—books from
the past which are still of interest to modern readers—on
subjects such as cooking, gardening, money, nature, travel,
sports, and history. Applewood Books are distributed by The
Globe Pequot Press of Old Saybrook, CT. For a free copy of
our current catalog, please write to: Applewood Books, c/o
The Globe Pequot Press, 6 Business Park Road, P.O. Box
833, Old Saybrook, CT 06475-0833.

10 9 8 7 6 5 4 3 2 1

Library of Congress Cataloging-in-Publication Data
Sanger, Margaret, 1879-1966.
      Happiness in marriage / by Margaret Sanger. —
Facsim. ed.
         p.   cm.
      Reprint. Originally published: New York: Brentano's,
1926.
      ISBN 1-55709-204-4 : $12.95
      1. Sex in marriage.   I. Title.
HQ31.S18   1993
646.7'8—dc20   92-42048
                                 CIP

TO THE NEW GENERATION
WHO SEEK HAPPINESS IN MARRIAGE
BASED ON TRUTH
THIS BOOK IS DEDICATED

CONTENTS

This book deals with the problems of normal sex love and marriage. It does not deal with sexual diseases or abnormalities. The course of true love does not run smoothly, truly says an old adage. Even aside from considerations of venereal diseases and such pitfalls, legitimate, married love is fraught with dangers. First essential a clean conception of sex. Failure of many modern marriages due to ignorance of sexual love. (1) Its central importance in life. (2) Its delicate instrument of expression. (3) Necessity for keeping alive the fire of romantic love. To understand growth, development and maturing of romantic sex love, we must go back to beginning of life; the building up of virility and beauty.

The dynamic energy of virility; youth and its problems; the conservation and storage of life energy; channeling and storing; reverence and respect for powers.

Courtship (for the young man): The importance of preliminaries; psychological factors; successful lovemaking. The value of courtship in building characters. The importance of good manners. Self-respect and reverence for loved one an essential in romantic love. Avoid petty negligence or thoughtlessness. The value of passion in life.

CONTENTS

INTRODUCTION

A SPOILED LIFE BECAUSE OF IGNORANCE

Love seeks mutuality, and grows by the sense and hope of responses.

—H. G. Wells.

California.

Dear Mrs. Sanger:

I have read your book, "What Every Girl Should Know," and can truthfully say I found it very helpful. But there is only one fault to find. I did not read it soon enough. I matured very late—at the age of 17. After I reached the age of puberty, I commenced going out with boys. I was very poor so could not have the pretty clothes so I took them from the young men I went with—giving myself in payment. Now here is the problem. The last young man I went with gave me a sickness. But I did not know this at the time. (I am now 24 years old).

Then I met the one man for me. We went steady for six months secretly of course as I will explain later. He proposed and I told him all concerning my past. He loved me enough to excuse it so we eloped leaving a note for my mother. We were married in San Francisco. About ten days afterward I found I had given him my sickness I did not know that I had the sickness until he told me. My husband still loves me and does not blame me. He lays the blame to my parents. They were old fashioned, strictly so. No young men were allowed to visit my home and I was not allowed to go out. The only way to go anywhere was to sneak out after the family was in bed. My mother was 45 years of age when I was born. She is now 69 years old. I don't know as it is helping matters any, but I want you

3

to know exactly how matters are. My mother is very religious. To go on—I was pretty popular and a good dancer and I do not wish to be vain but am telling the truth, much sought after. My dances were always taken. I could not keep my things at home so kept them at the home of my chum. This girl was the same only she had had no mother since the age of seven. She did all the work of the house and her father who was indifferent to what she did.

Now dear friend, what can I do. My husband loves babies and we are looking forward to the time when we will be able to have one but of course we can have none in our condition. I am willing to give all I have to my husband as I love him dearly and would willingly kill myself if it would make him well.

We live in a small town and have very little money. My husband works by the day and we cannot afford to go to a good doctor and we do not want it known that we are sick as we are very popular with people.

Let me hear from you as soon as possible and tell me to the best of your knowledge what is to be done. We would be very thankful. Anxiously awaiting your answer.

Mrs. R. B. K.

INTRODUCTION

THIS book aims to answer the needs expressed in thousands on thousands of letters to me for help in the solution of marriage problems. The suggestions and answers offered in each individual chapter are based upon the study and observation of these cases for a period of many years. I have been forcibly struck with the repetition and recurrence of the same questions, the same tragedies, the same problems in a large majority of these cases. On the basis of this experience I have assumed that these problems, to a greater or lesser extent, are present in most modern marriages. In this little book I offer solutions that are the outgrowth of observation of individual cases.

In seeking to solve any single problem of married life, we have often found that some new or unforeseen problem takes the place of the old one. Thus, as intelligent women seek to escape the trap of unwilling and enforced maternity to change their position from that of docile, passive child bearers to comrades and partners of their husbands, they realize the need of a more abundant and deeper love life. As they attain equality in professional and social relations, they become conscious of the need for equality and fuller expression in the more sacred intimacies of the marriage relation. Husbands as well as wives today realize the importance of complete fulfillment of love through the expression of sex. Unfortunately, due to the traditional conspiracy of silence in a phase of life in which more than anywhere else enlightenment is our crying need, marital happiness and lives are foredoomed to failure.

Light—more light is more necessary here than in any other of life's activities. The real and happy consummation of marriage between men and women cannot work any injury to morality. Nor can it destroy the institution of marriage. On the contrary, happiness in marriage—the complete union of body and mind—can only reinforce and strengthen the ties between man and woman. This is the only enduring solution to marriage problems. Only thus can we prevent the recurrence of those tragedies of marriage to which we have today as a nation become so cynically calloused and indifferent.

The question will inevitably arise—"Is not a book like this a danger to the morals of the young and unmarried?" No. Emphatically No. The young of today are demanding knowledge that will help them in life.

As I have two sons still in the adolescent age, it is my desire to spare them the failure and bitterness, disappointments, disillusions and heartaches that some of us of this generation have known. I want my sons to realize and to know what the past generation should have known on the threshold of life.

The great tragedy of today and of the past is that men and women have learned the great primary lessons of life too late. Let us do everything in our power to prevent among the rising generation the useless repetition of the tragedies of wrecked lives.

I believe that many mothers feel dissatisfied with the books that have been published because they lack the frankness and simplicity which should accompany the introduction of the sex subject.

Knowledge of sex truths frankly and plainly presented cannot possibly injure healthy, normal, young minds. Concealment, suppression, futile attempts to veil the unveilable—these work injury, as they seldom succeed and only render those who indulge in them ridiculous. For myself, I have full confidence in the cleanliness, the open-mindedness, the promise of the younger generation. Instead of seeking futilely to obstruct the creation of a new world, let us help them in their forward march into the future.

THE DESIRE FOR KNOWLEDGE

Minnesota.

I have just been reading your inspiring book on "Woman and the New Race". It is a wonderful explanation for a great many things, but it fails to answer so many questions, so I am taking the liberty of writing you personally, and begging you to answer some questions that are vital to my happiness. I am twenty years old, and although I have travelled about quite a bit I have led an extraordinarily sheltered life, I am beginning to believe. Until my mother was taken from me, I had no desire to associate with boys except as friends, and my mother never forbid me to have them in that way. But now that I have met the man I am going to marry in the spring, as soon as my school term is up, there are many things I feel I must know. I have had a shrinking feeling against sending for various books printed on the subject by physicians but I must do that if you can't help me. I don't know how this will strike you but the only person to whom I can talk about this is this boy. His knowledge is limited, but was gained in the very best way—from his mother and father. At first I felt that the urge I felt when I was with him and which I knew he had aroused within me, was something never to be mentioned. It developed, however, that he had understood and realized exactly how I felt, and guessed at my ignorance of it all. I don't believe I could have been as happy with him as I am if he had not told me that the feeling was as old as the human race and nothing to be ashamed of. Up to this time, I had thought that marriage meant loving one another and in some distant time having perhaps, one or two wonderful little children to help perpetuate

10

the race, and for us to love. But now, I know that there is this other phase of life which you refer to as the love life. At first I thought it must be some base passion, but I know it is not as we love each other more dearly than I had ever thought was possible. I know that this feeling will probably become greater after marriage, and as you say, will then be sanctioned by law. But—what can be done about it? It is evidently a very normal phase of almost every person's life, yet no light on the subject can be given publicly because of the law. I know I am over-stepping the bounds of convention and imposing on your patience by writing such a long letter, but you are the only person I can go to who really knows, and is intensely interested, and informed on her subject. I will wait very, very anxiously for a reply and a definite answer, if possible, to my question. If such an answer cannot be sent through the mails, is there any other suggestion you could make?

E. L. S.

CHAPTER I

THE FIRST STEP

' AND so they married and lived happily ever afterwards." Such is the conventional ending of most love stories. In life, however, the real love story does not end with marriage. It begins with it. Happiness is not the inevitable consequence of marriage. Marriage does not necessarily create happiness. Too often it destroys it. If husband and wife are to live joyously together, they must create their own happiness. Most people agree that happiness in marriage is often the exception rather than the rule. It is not a prize guaranteed with every marriage certificate. Even though bride and bridegroom be romantically in love with each other, they may find, after a few months of life together, that this mysterious reward has been withheld from them. They often discover that love is gradually fading. Married love died a long, lingering death. They awake to reality disillusioned, surprised to find themselves deprived of that abiding happiness they had expected.

This tragedy of modern marriage is usually the outgrowth of ignorance and misunderstanding. Happiness in marriage is not a matter of chance. It is a growth. Like all other living and growing organisms, it must first germinate, then strike root and then, after careful tending and cultivation, be brought to maturity. Only thus may it bloom and bear fruit. Sex attraction alone or the instinctive love of husband for wife and wife for husband is not enough. Self sacrifice is not enough. Romantic generosity is not enough. Fidelity is not enough. All these fine traits may enter into the marriage relationship, and yet, notwithstanding, marital happiness may be destroyed.

Fear and ignorance are the greatest destroyers of love. Fear alone will often kill the happiness that is born of real love. Therefore, where marriage is bound by fear and ignorance, there can be no happiness. The first essential in the establishment of happiness in marriage is the uprooting of fear and the banishing of sex ignorance. When this is done the foundation of happiness is laid.

Let us not forget that ignorance and fear

often assume the form of shame. Married love is possible when men and women have acquired a clean, healthy conception of sex, and through it a clean, wholesome fund of knowledge. In modern life, particularly in this country, the reproductive and sexual functions have been fenced off as mysterious facts, separate and distinct from the other activities of every-day life. Modesty has defeated itself in prurience and prudery. For women to remain in ignorance concerning the most important phase of their nature was until a few years ago considered good taste. Even biologists of the past generation ignored the facts of reproduction and sex as not intricately and organically connected with the well being of the individual and the race. Sex remained a deep, dark mystery, to be spoken of only in whispers, or not at all. This mystery was the cause of ignorance. Ignorance was the cause of disease and disease in its many forms was the cause of unhappiness and innumerable family tragedies.

The cost of this shameful sentimentality is too great. We cannot afford to remain in ignorance. Our own personal health is at stake. The future well being of the human race is at stake. We must learn to view sex and sex love as something other than physiological functions unrelated to the rest of our bodies and minds. Modern scientists are showing us that there is no part of our being that is not organically and intimately related to the love and sex life.

Romance based on ignorance cannot bear healthy fruit. In the past, when men and women were the victims of a huge conspiracy of silence concerning sex, experience was bought at a high cost. Young men were tacitly permitted to "sow their wild oats," venereal scourges resulted. Tragic and widespread and destructive as syphilis and gonorrhea are, spiritual destruction is even worse. Promiscuity, prostitution and disease destroy, sometimes forever, a clean and reverent attitude toward the physical sex relation. Pre-marital promiscuity has created in man an attitude of ruthless selfishness. More than any other single factor this has been destructive of mutual happiness in the lives of married people.

But women have, in the past, been too willing victims of this conspiracy of silence. Even today, with all our education, with all our organizations for social uplift, girls are brought up in absolute and fatal ignorance of the true meaning of the sexual function. To their normal, healthy curiosity the only answer has been that the sex instinct is in some mysterious way either a lewd, lascivious and unmentionable subject or too sacred and holy to mention.

Marriage based on a young man's experience without knowledge and a girl's ignorance without experience is foredoomed to inevitable failure. If love survives despite such an initial handicap, it proves its greatness. As a matter of fact, few marriages do. Divorces, separations, ruined lives, cynical husbands, hysterical wives, infidelities and all manner of family tragedies attest to the failure of the traditional approach to marriage. If they dared to give a frank answer, most men and women would tell you that love after marriage disappears and happiness is a gamble.

For marriages built upon the shifting sands of fear, shame and ignorance can never lead to happiness, yet if contracted with a frank recognition of the central importance of the beauty of sex in life, alike in its physiological, psychological and spiritual aspects, happiness becomes a glowing possibility. This is a buried treasure to be unearthed by true lovers. It may be imbedded in the rich soil of mutual respect and consideration. Carefully nurtured, it will strike deep roots in both lives, entwine and unite them together in ever-growing joy. It will grow, mature, bear fruit.

Few as they are, marriages of this type are nevertheless possible. To such unions we must look for guidance. Participants in happy relationships of this type are creators in the truest sense. Their intimate experience becomes a guide for all to follow. All the world loves such lovers. These are the creative artists pointing the way to spiritual awakening, that is possible to all men and women of the next generation, affecting all generations to come.

Sex educators today insist upon the so-called single standard of morality. The "wild oats" theory and its practice have proved ruinous. After years of effort, the educators have broken through the Chinese wall of silence erected by misguided prudery, and insist upon the necessity of purity and cleanliness of both parties in the marriage relation.

This is undoubtedly a step in the right direction, but let us not delude ourselves into believing that the single standard is a cure-all and end-all of sexual difficulties.

Such a practice may succeed in protecting our youth from the grosser evils of venereal infection and the dangers of promiscuity, but it does not touch the real problem of mating. No man or woman should leave to chance or the play of blind instinct, the most complex of all human ties. For even though young men and women bring to the marriage bed clean bodies and minds, they bring at the same time a lack of experience and understanding which may forever destroy the foundations of happiness. Even for those who believe the procreative act to be solely for the propagation of the race, it would be necessary to master and guide and have knowledge of the powerful instinct of sex.

Sex expression is not merely a propagative function, nor the satisfaction of an animal appetite. It should not be considered merely as a necessary evil preliminary to the production of a family. Sex expression, rightly understood, is the consummation of love, its completion and its consecration. Sex expression is an art. To become artists in love, men and women must learn to master and control the instruments by which this art is expressed.

These instruments are not merely the so-called sex organs, isolated and unrelated to the body or personality. If marriage is to be fully consummated, the entire body and spirit as units must participate in the union.

Think long and deeply over the importance of this truth. Until husband and wife have come to a realization of the necessity for complete union of body and spirit, happiness cannot grow out of the marriage relation. This union is possible only when both have acquired mastery of the physical instruments of expression. The body is not an enemy of the spirit. Our bodies are a visible expression. of our inner selves. Every factor, every gesture, every organ and function of our bodies is given us for the expression of our impulses, thoughts and desires. More than any other bodily act, sex expression is a sacred gift which awakens men and women to the innate beauty of life. We must learn to use this gift instead of misusing it. We must learn how to master the instrument of bodily expression so that passion is transmuted into poetry, so that life itself becomes lyric. In his grotesque attitude and use of sex in life the average man today is truly said to be like an orangoutang trying to play a violin. Discord instead of harmony has resulted.

Before reading the chapters which follow cleanse your mind of prurience and shame. Never be ashamed of passion. If you are strongly sexed, you are richly endowed. You possess the greatest and most valuable inheritance a human being can enjoy. To be strongly sexed means that the life force can suffuse and radiate through body and soul. It means radiant energy and force in every field of endeavor. It means driving power, ambition, attainment, but on condition that this great dynamic power be mastered and directed, stored and controlled, instead of dissipated and misspent. Without passion, love would be a flaccid, lifeless thing. Passion is the driving power of life. It cannot be denied, destroyed, or thrust aside. It must and it will find expression in some way—in destruction if its power be denied or not directed to creative ends. While it is a cruel master, it is also a willing slave.

Men and women have been endowed with

this dynamic energy which we name passion for the rounding out, the development, the fulfilling and the beautification of their natures. Those who deny it expression, who combat it, or who refuse to participate in it, cut themselves off from the zest and the poetry of life. They lead, narrow, warped, onesided lives. On the other hand, those who become the slaves of passion, or misuse it mainly through selfishness or in rebellion against the narrow traditions of the nineteenth and early twentieth centuries, also deprive themselves of greater development and attainment.

You men and women who stand at the threshold of maturity, learn to steer skillfully between the ascetic rocks and the sensual whirlpools. As George Meredith expresses it, "Onward to the creation of certain nobler races."

It is not enough to avoid the pitfalls of venereal disease, to trust to luck or blind instinct in the pursuit of happiness in marriage. It is not enough, great and invaluable as this gift is, to bring virility and passion to the nuptial bed. Clean bodies and minds you must bring, but romance, knowledge, poetry and art as well, and above all, keen anticipation and appreciation of the meaning of the most intimate and the most thrilling adventure life can offer you.

This is the first step towards happiness in marriage.

DEAR MRS. SANGER:

You have helped so many may be you can help me. I'm in love with a young man. It is the first man I have ever really loved (tho I have gone with a number and have been very good friends with them). Now we have had a plain talk I'm sure it would shock my mother but I believe it is best. He has never told me that he loves me nor I have never told him how much he means to me but he tells me that I arouse his passion that when we are together that his passion is so great he can hardly stand it. Tho, we have gone together over two years he has just recently told me this. He says he never was that way with any other girl and he is thirty and has gone with the girls for years. I'm not a flirt or flippey but what I want to know is what causes such passion. What is the reason. I'm not unduly passionate my self. I'm afraid to think of marrying him as I'm afraid the sex attraction is all he will ever have for me and that he will soon tire of that. A friend tells me that a marriage like that is the strongest. I never did allow familiarities but seems like his passion for me was always great. It will help me considerable if you will kindly tell me what causes such attraction and if marriage with a man like that would be satisfactory or likely to be happy. I have such a deep feeling and high regard for marriage. Thanking in advance I remain.

E. F.

CHAPTER II

BUILDING UP LIFE FORCES

"To everything there is a season, and a
Time to every purpose under the heaven."
—*Ecclesiasties III. I.*

ENDURING happiness in marriage cannot be won merely by the selection of the
right mate or the observation of certain rules
of sexual hygiene. Love is essential. Passion
is essential. Virility is essential. Mastery of
the instruments of expression is essential. But
if they have been wasted and dissipated in
premature and premarital profligacy, none of,
these essentials can be brought to marriage.

In this chapter, therefore, we must consider
the period of body-building, the conservation
and developing of life energies from infancy
to maturity.

In many respects the first period of life is
the most important. By the first period I
mean that which includes childhood, youth and
early manhood. In primitive and uncivilized
people maturity comes at a very early age.

Reproduction follows swiftly. The new generation likewise rapidly passes through the life cycle. One generation follows another in rapid succession—childhood, youth, old age all come too swiftly. Individuals are consequently seldom able to attain a full development, and consequently in those races in which the life cycle is short and swift, are backward in individual development and in their civilization as well.

This same process may be seen in our own country. We see many boys and girls who cannot or will not remain young. Prematurely they rush into life's most serious experiences. Precociously and thoughtlessly they leap into marriage and often become old before their time. They waste their inner energies; scatter their powers; glide over the surface of life, instead of conserving their forces to prepare for intense and mature experience. In the end, those young men and women who clamor for immediate and premature sex expression cheat themselves of that lasting happiness all men and women crave.

Childhood, youth and early manhood are not merely given to us as periods of preparation. It is a grave mistake to hurry through them.

Youth must not try to cut them short. The greatest thinkers today assert that life can be most fully realized only by the prolongation of this period of preparation for maturity by the conservation of early powers.

The foremost educators no longer aim to turn children into little men and women, but rather to develop the full possibilities of childhood, to bring out all its hidden potentialites. Similarly with adolescence, youth and early manhood. People try to make short-cuts through these periods, or to dispense with them altogether, instead of growing and developing through them. They find themselves, nevertheless, forever chained to the unfulfilled desires of those cheated and stunted periods.

Some years ago a girl who had married at the age of fourteen came to see me. The first thing we knew this girl-wife was playing marbles with my children in the garden. "Married women don't play marbles," exclaimed my shocked laundress. "I would rather play than be married," the girl-wife retorted.

Many women of thirty or even forty go back when there is the opportunity to the innocent gaieties and pleasure they have missed during their adolescent period. They were thrust at too early an age into the more serious realities of married life. "My husband is kind, but he doesn't understand me, we are so un- congenial," one of these women confessed to me. "I like to go to dances and parties and have innocent flirtations. I like pretty clothes and admiration. My husband cannot under- stand why at my age I am so frivolous." This woman had been married at the age of seven- teen, and the legitimate and innocent pleasures of adolescence had been denied her. As ma- turity developed, these instincts clamored for expression.

A man was sentenced to prison at the age of twenty-one. When he was released he was a middle-aged man. He resumed his emotional development at the point where it had been cut off when he was sent to prison. He desired to associate with girls of the age attractive to him before his conviction. Altogether in every other respect he was mentally mature. In fact, this man of fifty-two eventually married a girl of fifteen.

Innumerable instances of arrested emotional development caused by forcing young men and girls at too early an age into the problems of maturity and marriage, come readily to mind.

Both physically and mentally, the first twenty years of life, and preferably the first twenty-three years of life, should be the period of upbuilding and conservation.

The whole process of building up the body, its bones, muscles, sinews, nerves; in fact, its very architecture is dependent upon the internal secretions and is intricately connected with the sexual system.

During the period of body-building, especially between the ages of twelve and twenty-three, the coördination of those secretions, hormones or chemical messengers absorbed directly into the blood stream are modeling the bone structure and the fine symmetry of body that makes for virility and beauty. In this vital and all-important process of body-building, the sex glands play a part of equal importance with the other ductless glands, the importance of which, modern science tells us, cannot be overestimated. The symmetry, the strength, the vigor of the body, with its bones, its sinews, its delicately coördinated muscles, its internal organs (heart, lungs, liver, etc.) is dependent upon the harmonious activity of these glands.

To tamper with the sex organs, to interfere

with their development, to dissipate or to divert these secretions which should be contributing their chemical powers to the upbuilding of virile and beautiful bodies, means actually to throw the whole process of construction out of balance. Even though the body-building continues, a discord not always noticed by unobservant eyes, has entered, and the full, complete, and well-rounded development, and the full maturity and harmony of physical and mental powers by this interference are sometimes forever defeated.

All activity—mental and physical—during this period, when the foundations of life are being laid and the structure of the body is being erected, should be determined by this process. No one can go back and build his life anew. The mistakes men make during the teens must somehow be paid for. Too often they are paid for in the thirties and forties. Whoever begins to waste life at an early age, shall inevitably find that his bank account of virility, strength and passion is exhausted when he most needs it.

Human bodies are both dynamos and motors. Before the nervous and emotional power can be directed and expended, it must be created and stored up. This is what is going on for the first twenty or twenty-three years of life. The more vital power stored up in bones, muscles, nerves and sinews (instead of dissipated), the greater the force of its expenditure during maturity, the later its use, the longer the period of virility. To store away vitality and sex energy in youth means a greater power and fuller use of it in maturity.

A fruit tree planted in rocky, poverty-stricken soil, cannot produce its full quota of fruit. It cannot store up nor drink in the necessary elements necessary to produce a full harvest. It withers and dies. So it is with a human life. Before we can mature and produce the fruits of maturity, we must attain a full growth.

There is a time when love and sex expression become of primary importance to our well being. But before that period arrives, in order to prepare fully for this consecrating experience, the young must learn to refrain from lesser sex experiences and temptations which may, and often do, render impossible the greater drama of love of which all humans are desirous.

Each process, each period of life, has its own

reason. Life is a chain, each period a link. Each link dependent upon the preceding for its power and strength. We cannot hurry through, neglect or shorten them. The growing period, the controlling and storing-up period, the self-creative period is not only beautiful; it is a necessary preliminary to that which follows. Sex energy and passion is not only controlled but stored up, for without this great latent passion, this deep reservoir, passion cannot at the great moment express its power nor the overwhelming poetry of life find full expression.

"If you don't start life with a head of steam, you won't get far," says Lord Dawson of Penn. Let us remember that this head of steam does not just happen. It is generated, stored up in a miraculous way acknowledged and partially understood only by scientists, but ready to be converted, as the mysterious miracle of sex love, into ambition.

COURTSHIP FOR THE MAN

DEAR MADAM:—

I would like you to give me good information or advice about girls so that I may talk to them. I am lone my father and mother are dead over ten years and my sisters live in St. Louis and Memphis.

I am 27 years old not married I never go with girls. Never talk with them nor call on them but one. They never invite me to dance party. I don't understand why. This is my home town and I love it. I do not want to go to City to find girls company.

I do not want to ask town boys for advice as they put me in wrong way. I would like to work out the problem myself.

I do hope you will help me.

J. B.

CHAPTER III

COURTSHIP—FOR THE MAN

"Let them have a period of courtship, for it
is my desire and will that true love should
forever precede marriage" . . . —*Brahma*.

THE importance of courtship cannot be
overemphasized. Wooing not only possesses its own beauty, but it is a step that
should never be neglected in the foundation of
a happy marriage. It should not be looked
upon as a troublesome preliminary encouraged
only by custom and tradition, but like infancy,
childhood and youth, this period is a necessary
and beautiful one in any well-rounded, developed life.

An ardent wooer is most apt to be a successful husband. A negligent, thoughtless, or
careless wooer very often is unable to bring
happiness to any woman.

Yet, skillful art to woo is not a God-given
gift showered upon some fortunate young men
and denied to the rest. Nature has wisely provided normal and healthy young men with the

rudiments of this art. Given the necessary interest and ardor awakened by the process known as "falling in love," a young man need only use his intelligence eloquently to express this fine impulse.

First of all, he must recognize that thought-lessness is the first barrier to love. If he thinks only to satisfy his own wishes, he can scarcely hope to awaken in his sweetheart enduring love. The girl may be partially in love with this youth, but if on repeated occasions she is hurt by unconcealed or ill-concealed selfish acts, she is bound to be disappointed.

Thoughtlessness, ordinarily, takes the form of selfishness. The successful wooer must therefore learn to think first of the wishes of his beloved and do all in his power to fulfill her hidden desires. His early experiences in juvenile or adolescent courtship may form the basis of his experience in the all-important rôle of marriage.

Remember that games and sports of every kind develop the sense of good sportsmanship and fair play. These are part of the foundations of behavior. In mature life the rules of the game are essential also for the life of love.

Nevertheless, when the young man falls seriously in love, when the blind, imperious and driving grip of sex attraction holds him, his early training in self-control must help him to become its master and not its slave. This instinct is powerful. It seeks only its own satisfaction. It is a primitive, ferocious, consuming force that so often drives the young lover to actions which would appear selfish. Many young men, fine fellows and admirable in all other fields of life, often fail to master this imperious instinct; thereby defeating their own purpose and happiness.

This is the real cause of so many elopements, runaway marriages, misalliances. Many are said to "fall in love with a pretty face." Passion gets the upper hand, and they choose as a mate some girl manifestly unfitted by character, training and personality to become a life mate, although her very qualities might make her by taste and temperament a most suitable wife for some other man. Not all runaway marriages are failures, but like most reckless acts, the risk is great, and when one realizes that one may be gambling upon one's whole future happiness, the young man and the young woman as well should stop and think before leaping into the unchartered sea of premature matrimony.

Every marriage should be skillfully launched. The period of wooing is the wise provision of nature and custom by which both youth and girl are permitted to discover the hidden qualities in the character of the other, qualities which mean infinitely more in the building and creating of married happiness than conventional skin-deep beauty or handsomeness.

For the young man, wooing must be a great adventure. It is a voyage of discovery and exploration. He discovers the hidden beauties in the character of the one he loves concealed behind the curtain of her modesty, or even unknown to her. He discovers her innocent whims, her buried wishes. Then, by compliments, little gifts or thoughtful acts, he brings to her attention by a series of surprises the results of this voyage.

Long before physical love between them is possible, there may be a psychic or spiritual communion between two young persons. This psychic prelude is absolutely necessary as a prerequisite for successful love-making on a physical plane. Psychic and spiritual unity is essential—otherwise love would remain on the level of a physiological function.

Inhibited and restrained by the false restrictions of so-called polite society, too many repressed young men take up the task of love-making in too tame and effete a style. "Faint heart ne'er won fair lady," says the old adage.

I have perhaps over-emphasized the danger of becoming a slave to passion, but one must not forget that there must be passion. There must be an imperious, driving force in back of all wooing. It should never be permitted to sink to the boresome fulfillment of a certain number of weekly or monthly calls, tiresome, restrained participation in ordinary social functions. Romance, to live, must not be caged in the atmosphere of tame domesticity, nor deprived of the opportunity to soar.

To the young man, therefore, who would woo successfully, I urge these suggestions:

First, Dramatize your love;

Second, Carry into action the generous impulses inspired and awakened by your beloved;

Third, Be aggressive. It is the rôle of love to act; be fearless but at the same time be chivalrous, for aggressiveness without respect is brutal and offensive.

But this does not mean that the lover should not "act out" his ardor. When I counsel you to dramatize your love, I mean that instead of seeking satisfaction in reveries, day dreams, or morbid fancies, you should seek to awaken and hold the interest of the girl of your heart by a continuous series of surprises, unexpected meetings, gifts, tokens and evidences that indicate to her that she is uppermost and supreme in your thoughts.

Many young lovers today are too likely to assume that they can easily hold the interest of the girl they love. They take too much for granted. This is the reason so many love affairs die a slow, lingering death. The youth may be able to arouse the interest of a girl, but how long can he hold it?

Remember that the majority of girls, no matter how completely mistresses of themselves they may at first appear, are often filled with misgivings concerning their own attractiveness and desirability. Usually girls are more acutely aware of what they consider their bad points than they are conceited over their good points.

The adroit and intelligent lover must seek to reawaken in the girl a sense of her own value,

her own worthiness, her own charm. The
wooer thus creates in his beloved a sense of
self-esteem and happiness. He is creating a
hitherto inexperienced elation, a warmth which
brings the color to the girl's cheeks, an ecstasy
which makes her eyes bright, so that, in brief,
love actually does work a strange miracle. The
girl, in many cases, becomes almost as beautiful as the wooer believes her to be. Love may
cure, as some have claimed, and it is no less
certain that it brings a new beauty to the
beloved.

By such means as these the young woman is
made conscious that she also possesses the
mysterious power to inspire love, to awaken
desire. By words, looks, glances half concealed, the girl is brought by the adroit lover
to the satisfying realization that her good
points by far outnumber her defects. Beauty
lies in the eye of the beholder, and the real
wooer must awaken in his beloved the realization that she is charming and to him as desirable as she would like to be.

The average girl is a Cinderella at heart.
The man who would be a successful wooer
must re-enact the rôle of the Prince.

There is, after all, a poet hidden in the heart

of every ardent wooer. The poetry inspired by love need not always be expressed in words, but the lover must aim to awaken the girl's latent interest in the infinite variety of the world, increase her zest and enjoyment of life. He must learn to invest the simplest everyday activities of living with a keener pleasure. Under his magic spell, life, which heretofore may have been drab and monotonous to her, takes on a more vivid color and beauty.

A poor young man, just starting in the great battle for a living and economic independence, may here object that such a courtship may lead him into debt, but this need not be so. Costly gifts and expensive entertainments showered on a young girl are not necessary. It is not the amount or the quantity of gifts that wins a girl's heart. For unless they are the outward expression of a fine inner love, they can mean little to the girl who is worth winning.

On the other hand, the man in love, finding economic barriers, actually may be aided in his siege by being forced to develop ingenuity by planning innumerable inexpensive, unexpected surprises, even by adding a touch of secrecy to his courtship and thus making it more of an adventure and more thrilling to both.

I even go so far as to claim that love is often strengthened when confronted by obstacles. For each obstacle overcome, each obstruction surmounted, increases the man's confidence in himself. A prize lightly won is rarely highly valued.

There are innumerable possibilities in gestures which the skillful wooer will make use of to express his thoughtfulness and ardor. He will find out the favorite color, the preferred perfume, the favorite flower of the girl he loves, as well as all of her caprices and whims.

So many men make the mistake of concerning themselves too exclusively with their own emotions, their own instincts, their own pleasures, their own needs. But the successful lover, on the other hand, concentrates all of his attention on the woman of his choice. His whole effort in courtship is to awaken the woman he desires to the realization that she is essential to his well being, as necessary as sunlight and fresh air. To him she becomes a supreme being, respected and worshipped. With every word, every gesture and act he

aims to lift this love out of the realm of reality
into that of romance, or, better still, he trans-
mutes her ordinary, everyday world with the
beauty of romance and love.

And if he fail? If the girl whom he has
selected as the object of his love be fickle, or
capricious, or unable through some innate de-
ficiency or restriction, to reciprocate his ardor,
is all of love's labor lost? To this there is but
one answer—No! There is profound truth in
the saying, " 'Tis better to have loved and lost
than never to have loved at all." To woo, seriously, desperately, ardently and dramatically
—this in itself, irrespective of the final outcome—victory or defeat—is one of life's most
noble, valuable and far-reaching experiences.

The great danger of the disappointed lover
lies in the fact that he may succumb to the
temptation of becoming a self-pitying cynic
concerning women. If he has courted her
ardently, adroitly, skillfully, tenderly, and
nevertheless is faced finally with defeat, this
experience will, notwithstanding, have taught
him much. It will have heightened and intensified his appreciation of the meaning of
life. It will have taught him the significance
of pain and defeat—great teachers, both. But

the very ecstasy of the experience he has gone through, the tonic effect of his enjoyment, the increased zest he has felt in the simple, every-day pleasures of living, will remain in the young man's memory. They will remain long after the pain of defeat has been forgotten, and it will be the memory of this first great love affair, even if perchance it has not led to a happy marriage, that will spur him on to new conquest, make him a more ardent, more skillful and inevitably a more successful husband.

There are no set rules or regulations for courtship. There are no signposts leading straight to the heart of a woman. Each love must create anew the rules of life's great game. It does not matter so much how difficult its rules are, provided only that both play it fair and square, on the level and above board.

The young man will remember that the keenest pleasure is in the pursuit, and let the young woman never forgot that what is easily won is lightly prized.

Courtship, in conclusion, must be adventurous, daring, exciting, romantic. The great danger in this day is not that it be too recklessly romantic, but that it be too tamely accepted, too anemic, too lifeless. The woman pursuing, the man passively accepting.

Many love affairs die of inanition. They never mature because of inhibitions, restrictions, suppressions and timid shames. When you fall in love, put life and joy into that love. Give yourself grandly to each stage of its journey. Do not be afraid to take the plunge in matrimony when you are sure of your love.

For love stimulates the whole glandular system, releases into the body a fresh supply of energy, breaks through the old inhibiting and hindering fears, sweeps aside narrow, prim and priggish ideas of life's values, brings new spring to the step, fresh color to the cheeks, depth and sparkle to the eye. Love taps an unsuspected and inexhaustible supply of energy which the young lover may convert into ambition and achievement. That is why all the world loves a lover and that is why men and women must learn to remain in love, even though married.

Dear Mrs. Sanger:

I am a young girl of 20 years and am going to marry soon. I have been hesitating for many months just for the reason that he is in the hospital, having been gassed in the army.

I love children very much and would not think of a home that was not blessed with them but under the circumstances, with my husband in his present state, I do not think it just right for me to go ahead and bring a little one into this world who might suffer the consequences. I have talked this matter over with him and he just says we can trust to luck about that but I just cannot see it as he does.

I purchased your book "Woman and the New Race" and read it and I thought you could help me in this matter since I have no one to talk it over with. I will be a young bride and I realize my ignorance on this subject and I am in perfect health now and would like to remain so.

I am educated and have my own way to make in this world. My future husband does not understand why I do not rush right on into marrying him and this is what has been bothering me all the time. The doctors say he will be well in another two years and we have been waiting so long that we have decided to marry now.

Mrs. Sanger if you can advise me, I would appreciate it very much and would only consider it as motherly advice. Thanking you I am

B. G. S.

CHAPTER IV

COURTSHIP—FOR THE GIRL

FOR the girl who stands at the threshold of life the period of courtship is even more important than for the young man. For centuries motherhood, not marriage, has been the chief function of mating. There is reason to expect that most normal women will continue to seek self-development and self-expression in the fields of marriage as well as motherhood.

Therefore it is essential that every girl in her late teens and early twenties should use all her intelligence and insight to develop herself mentally, emotionally and physically. Not that she should aim merely to prepare herself for the "marriage market," but she owes it to herself to appear and to live at her best.

No matter how limited her income today is, it is possible for every girl to make the most of her natural endowments. This requires study and attention and perhaps advice from some trusted, confidential friend.

Beauty is not the monopoly of a few girls

upon whom all gifts have been showered. Nature has endowed every woman with certain powers of attraction. Every woman is attractive in some way. No woman is attractive to all men. But every woman can make herself attractive to some men, and this is as it should be.

Certain things are essential to all. No beauty, no prettiness, no attractive qualities can you afford to neglect.

In the very first place, to all women health and hygienic cleanliness are absolutely essential. Over-confident in their power to attract admiration, many young girls become negligent in this respect. Such negligence must immediately be corrected.

It is within the power of every girl and young woman nowadays to develop and to keep radiantly fresh her natural charms. If she fails to do this, no amount of money spent on clothes, jewels, or superficial trinkets can possibly make her any more attractive to eligible young men.

In the first place, she must keep her body fresh and clean, free from the odors of perspiration and preventing, through daily care, the possibility of any unpleasantness in this respect. This is a delicate yet tremendously important problem of feminine hygiene which must be solved, not by a general rule, but by each girl personally.

Much of a girl's freshness and attractiveness depends upon proper diet and digestion and the healthy functioning of the processes of digestion and elimination—the stomach and the bowels. A fine skin and complexion cannot be kept if the stomach is disordered by careless eating and an overindulgence in starches and sweets. Chronic constipation is an enemy to beauty. A sweet, wholesome breath depends to a great extent upon these vital processes of elimination. Every intelligent girl will realize the importance of the internal as well as the external care of the body. Less active and indulging in fewer sports than men, girls are more often victims of constipation.

The care of the teeth and mouth must become a part of the daily routine. The proper care of the hands and fingernails is also a necessary routine. The hair, which is properly called a woman's crowning glory, must be thoroughly cared for, brushed and groomed daily if it is to retain its glossy life and beauty.

The coiffure is an art no longer neglected by American women, and today, when its importance is being fully realized, there is an infinite variety of styles, bobs and cuts that have proven a Godsend to many.

In the matter of dress, girls have a far greater opportunity for charm and attractiveness than ever before. By the use of intelligence, common sense and good taste, even the girl of limited income can choose a wardrobe of great attractiveness.

Every article will be chosen by the sensible girl, not because it happens to be the latest fad or fashion (and may be particularly unsuited to her individual figure and complexion), but with a careful attention to the problem of whether it enhances and "brings out" her good points. Each girl must learn to develop a style and individuality in dressing, choosing clothes and colors which accentuate her type, at the same time exercising great care that she does not render herself cheaply conspicuous. Men are proud to be seen in the company of girls who are striking and stylish; but most men are embarrassed by girls who are loud in manner, whether it be in voice or in clothes and complexion.

The care of the body, both outwardly and inwardly, the bathing and thorough cleanliness of all of its orifices, give the girl an assurance of sweet-smelling cleanliness which gives her an invaluable assurance and confidence in her own power of attractiveness. Her mind is no longer weighed down by nervous doubts concerning her physical defects or deficiencies. Her appearance is no longer a matter of chance nor merely of a perishable prettiness, but it bespeaks intelligence and character as well. A wholesome selfishness in this matter of personal appearance and style is healthy and normal in a girl who does not care to leave her life and future happiness entirely to chance.

The girl who can study herself and use discrimination and judgment in the care of her body and in the selection of a wardrobe, will by this exercise of intelligence be enabled to judge and discriminate between the types of suitors who are attracted to her.

Before the girl has found the man of her choice, there is a period that is important in her development, and yet is one of danger and uncertainty. It is during this period that the

girl must discover her own strength and her
own weaknesses.

During this period the attractive girl—and
I insist here that all girls possess natural powers of attractiveness which they themselves
must develop—the attractive girl finds herself,
in all classes of society, interesting to several
types of men. Some will be attentive merely
on the basis of good fellowship. There are
other boys, immature, unsettled, unsure of
their financial or economic position. There are
still other men who are ready and willing to
drift into any sort of relation possible, who
have a horror of assuming any of the more
serious responsibilities of life, and who are
aimless and vacillating in their intentions with
women.

Then there is a most dangerous and sinister
group—men and boys who are at heart gang-
sters, whether it be of a country club gang or
one which congregates at street corners. Both
to the sheltered debutante of society and to the
self-respecting girl who reliantly goes forth to
earn her own living, men of this type are not
to be encouraged. The chief aim of this sex
pirate is to return to his gang and boast of
his conquest of some girl and of the favors

he has won. Make no mistake about this: he tells of his intimacies, how far he has been able to go with the girl, and what chances others have for the same privilege. Such men have absolutely no respect for the girl who gives herself freely to them. In his mind, such a girl is merely a substitute for the prostitute whose price he cannot pay.

Girls in sheltered homes, closely chaperoned, may not frequently meet men of this type. But girls in business pursuits who work in stores, shops and factories, are thrown constantly in contact with such men She may redeem him from his sinister habits. But she can do so only by awakening in his mind a respect for her, not by succumbing to his suggestions or desires.

Finally, there is the man who falls seriously in love with the girl. He may be a man who has been an old friend, a companion, or an absolute stranger. Whether this flame be love at first sight or not makes little difference. Or perhaps there is the man with whom you, the girl, fall seriously in love.

This is the awakening, the new consciousness within yourself that you are in love, that you want with all your heart and soul this one man as your mate. If you sense that this deep feeling is returned, so much the better. If this man, who in your eyes differs from all other men, shows signs,—and there are innumerable ways of finding out—of wanting you in return, it is of the greatest importance that you be mistress of the situation.

At this point courtship begins. And in this important experience the girl no less than her suitor must play an active and all-important rôle. The final outcome of the game depends more upon the wooed than upon the wooer.

Many a possible romance and marriage have been thwarted by too passive an attitude or too hasty an acceptance on the part of the girl.

To awaken a desire, to nourish it, to cultivate it, to direct it,—this, Balzac has written, is a poem in itself. It is the poetry of courtship. It is the duty no less of the young woman than of the suitor.

If the initial friendship and good-fellowship upon which the intimacy between the suitor and the girl is founded is to be converted and ripened into the deeper feeling of enduring love, the girl must aim to awaken in the heart of the wooer a fine respect for her as a human being.

His desire will increase if she makes it impossible for him to take her interest for granted. Uncertainty is a greater stimulant to his interest than possession. Concealment is one of the most natural and legitimate of woman's arts. The suitor's interest is held and deepened by his effort to find out if the girl of his choice is really in love with him.

Do not play with his affection. But at the same time do not forget that the pursuit is a necessary link in the chain; and no matter how delighted you are that this man may be your mate, avoid premature consent. Remember again that a prize lightly won is not highly valued.

For the woman as well as the man the period of courtship or wooing demands a distinct technique. There is an art of being wooed as well as one of wooing.

Too many young women today have forgotten this. They forget that Nature and tradition have decreed that Man shall be the wooer, the pursuer, the huntsman. Man is the aggressor, and there is a profound psychological reason for the rightness of this view.

If the woman is clever enough to elude charmingly this pursuit, she becomes instrumental in intensifying his desire, in deepening his attraction in holding his interest.

It is therefore one of the first lessons for women to learn in the art of love; to be playfully elusive. She must respond to the advances of the man of her choice, but she must not respond too rapidly, too completely, too prematurely. She must remember that adventurous primitive man does not value highly an easy capture.

Desire is generated in the pursuit. The more venturesome the chase, the greater the vicissitudes overcome, the thrill of uncertainty, in brief, the whole prelude of anticipation, makes the lover set a greater value and interest on the object of his passion.

Today many women have forgotten this. And in neglecting to learn the elements of an art that is essentially feminine, in failing to realize the two-fold nature of courtship, they are disappointed in the lukewarm interest displayed by the wooer.

Uncertainty stimulates the wooer's interest. This, however, does not mean that even in the period of ardent wooing, sincerity and honesty should be cast aside. Quarrels, which to many may seem inevitable, should never be permitted to deepen or become anything more than superficial incidents of the courtship.

Thoughtless cruelty may kill or deaden forever an enduring love. Even though the lovers may be brought together again by mutual forgiveness, the wound remains. It may poison or infect the entire relationship.

The love of the majority of men is deepened and strengthened by resistance. It puts them on their mettle, gives them the necessary obstacles to overcome, and puts them to the test. The man who is easily defeated or willingly accepts disappointment is hardly the man who makes a good husband. Especially in the early days of courtship, it is the duty of the woman to aim to bring out the strength and courage of the suitor, not his childish weakness.

Just as the lover must seek to dramatize his love by a series of pleasant surprises and unexpected incidents, so, too, must the girl aim to discover the real man beneath the love by putting his character to unexpected tests.

Her aim from the beginning of courtship to the day when she finally consents to become his wife, should be to prevent this intimate and thrilling relationship from sinking to the level of the commonplace. Never permit your favors to become matter of fact.

The first requisite is to win this man's respect. Having won it, you must retain it, but without resorting to the crude weapons of coldness or affectation. It would be the utmost tactlessness to assert your own superiority by correcting his faults or calling his attention to personal defects in dress or manners. On the other hand, the clever girl may suggest to her swain certain changes in dress or deportment in a manner that will not offend him, and at the same time make her dearer to his heart. Do not criticize and find fault. Nagging is immoral. Encourage and stimulate to greater achievement by appreciation and respect.

Familiarity breeds contempt, rightly warns an old adage. This is especially true during the days of courtship. Therefore never cheapen this relationship, whatever its outcome may be, by undue faultfinding familiarity. Make it worthy and dignified, as you should make all human contacts.

A certain dignified reserve does not mean that you must coldly deprive yourself of any of the real pleasures of happy youth. But the girl should not forget that during the days of courtship the whole foundation of a lifelong relationship is being built. Good manners, politeness, courtesy, respect, and dignity are more necessary in these more intimate relationships than are involved in the relations of acquaintances or friends.

The highest compliment a man can pay a woman is to ask her to become his wife. Anything less is an experiment. Either it reveals his inability or his unwillingness to accept responsibility, or his fundamental selfishness in love. At any rate it bespeaks his unconscious confession that his love is not of the marrying kind. To enter such a relation is most likely to be a costly experience for a girl just entering maturity.

There is a wholesome reaction today against prudishness and priggishness in youth. This is indeed a healthy sign. But there is another danger in the swing of the pendulum to the opposite extreme. Laxity in speech and behavior, roughness and rudeness of manner, is not pleasing to men, rough and uncultured though they themselves may be. The noisy, conspicuous girl who in a group or party is seeking always to attract attention to herself is usually in this very act confessing her failure to hold the interest she so flamboyantly seeks to arouse. She only attracts to herself the same type of response.

The girl who is elusive, whose manner suggests that beneath a quiet exterior she is concealing qualities of strength and more endearing charms is bound to attract men of more sterling worth, who themselves have learned deeper and truer values of life, who seek in a woman finer and more profound beauty than a cheap and gawdy exterior, which so often conceals an empty head.

Gossip and questionable stories are incongruous and unsuitable for any girl's conversation, and create a bad impression with men, even though they may tolerate them. Nevertheless, such talk inevitably lowers the girl's moral standard in the eyes of her male companions. If she indulges in or tolerates loose coarse language concerning phases of life all humans should respect and reverence, the whole exalted tone of romantic lovemaking is vulgarized, and an element of cheapness and discord enters into a relationship that should be kept clean and poetic.

The younger generation today too often

confuses haste with frankness. With the decay of etiquette and advent of the new freedom of expression, haste and hurry, tactless frankness and bad manners in all phases of life, there can be little doubt that courtship is becoming one of the lost arts. But it is an art upon which most of the enduring happiness and stability of subsequent married life depends. It must not only be recaptured, but developed, refined and recognized as of primary and central importance in the technique of love.

The period of wooing is therefore the most beautiful as well as the most important in the lives of the young men and young women. It corresponds to the springtime of the year, and young love is like the young plant bursting through the soil. The young lover may for the first time awaken the young woman to the realization of her blind impulses, may unveil for her the mystery and the intensity of love. Small wonder that this has been the eternal theme in art, music and literature. Love embodied in a woman means a rebirth for the lover.

When at last the suitor has made a proposal of marriage, the girl doubtless has already considered her reply and should, nevertheless, continue mistress of the situation. She should have satisfied herself as to his character, that he is pleasing to her physically as well as mentally; that his virtues overweigh his faults; and that she is ardently in love with him.

If she does not believe they are suited to each other, she must have the courage and the honesty to reject him. Such a rejection, no matter how painful at the moment, will prevent the future and tragic unhappiness in two lives.

If on the other hand she forsees a community of love and interest, she can without reservation, accept the proposal and announce her engagement.

Michigan.

DEAR MRS. SANGER:

May I convide in you? for I dare not talk to my mother the way I am about to write to you. She would not understand.

I am engaged to be married in June, but dread it, as we can hardly control ourselves now, what would it be then? Can you help me please?

Is sexual intercourse wicked, if children are not wanted? I believe this is one of the worse evils of today. Is there anything one can do to prevent it? I don't mean to question God's ways, but do you know any help for "secret sin."

Could you suggest the best book for my purpose? I feel most too bold in sending this letter to you, but one must convide in somebody, and I thought you could help me if anyone could. Why were we made to want to indulge in that, only for our own pleasures, when children are not wanted. Why couldn't sexual intercourse happen only when it was meant to be. Is it because of sin?

That's why instead of looking forth with joy to next June, I wish the months would drag along until then, because it may mar our happiness as I have always looked upon this as a sin.

D. E. C.

CHAPTER V

ENGAGED

EXCHANGE of promises and the assurance of mutual love usher in the period of engagement. These are days of elation, excitement and exaltation. The period of the engagement is one of happy anticipation and joyful preparation.

At the same time it is a period of great danger. Impulses must be controlled by intelligence and foresight. This period leads the lovers one step nearer marriage. It is a period of greater intimacy, greater self-revelation, and more thorough knowledge of each other.

The greatest temptation for many engaged couples is to cast aside all discretion, all reticence, and actually to assume an attitude of familiarity which is almost identical with that of many married couples, the only reservation being the physical consummation of marriage.

It is true that the custom of the betrothal (or engagement) should permit the suitor and the beloved to establish a greater intimacy than that acquired during the period of courtship. But the engagement must never be considered as a sort of trial marriage with one important factor missing.

Dignity, reverence and respect for each other are more essential during this critical period than at any other. For during the engagement the habits of mutual courtesy and thoughtfulness must strike root. If they are not permitted to, through faultfinding or laxity of relations, the subsequent marriage will not be founded on a satisfactory basis and is bound to fail or to sacrifice one or both of the contracting parties to intolerable misery and unhappiness.

Among young girls and young men today there has arisen a free and easy laxity of relationship. Modesty as it was understood in the past century has disappeared. A greater freedom in speech has arisen, a freedom which sometimes degenerates into license. Although they may refrain from going "the limit," sexual liberties are indulged in by certain misguided couples.

Quite aside from all considerations of morality, the experience derived from such practices is not great enough to risk the sacrifice of true and enduring love. Their price is paid from the treasury of self-respect and mutual love.

Dignity, respect, reverence and romance are often destroyed by one false step along the path of physical indulgence. Such practices often result in broken engagements, and the unhappy humiliation of the girl who has permitted them. Even though the engagement continue and marriage ensue, she is often reminded of the favors previously given—making for suspicion and jealousy—the healthy reciprocity that should be maintained has been upset and an element of discordant moral weakness has poisoned the romance of betrothal.

The greatest danger which lies in wait during the engagement is the destruction of this spirit of romance. Intimacy may unconsciously be dragged down to the level of vulgar familiarity. Through thoughtlessness and lack of foresight destructive quarreling may be indulged in. The man and girl who indulge in quarrels begin to look at each other no longer with the eyes of love, but with suspicion, jealousy and criticism. And what is temporarily lost by such a practice is difficult, and often impossible, to regain.

The girl may begin to doubt the wisdom of her choice. The question arises in her mind: "Do I really love him?" She cannot make up her mind. She is torn between the desire to marry and to have all that her fiancé offers, and the desire to wait and to hope for someone else. She may be proud of his looks and his love for her. But with continued observation she may be annoyed and irritated by unpleasant or careless habits. She may discover to her dismay that his love for her has not wrought the miracle she had hoped for. His table manners, which she had never noticed in the first flush of romance, she may now discover to be hurried, awkward and crude. There may be dandruff on his collar and spots on his coat. There may be certain personal habits seemingly unimportant, but which are none the less irritating to a fastidious and romantic girl—unclean fingernails, teeth, etc., picking at the teeth, nose or ears, all sorts of unconscious movements or gestures which should never have arisen and which in all events should be immediately corrected. Slight as they may seem, they may cause in the girl a secret shame.

Because of the tremendous importance of these seemingly unimportant things, the suitor should make doubly certain that in every respect he is physically and personally attractive to the girl of his choice.

There should be no carelessness in his attire. It costs little to be well groomed in body and immaculate in dress. Attention to such details aids in making the meetings and the tryst exceptionable and romantic events, not mere workaday habits.

The engaged man should never lose sight of the fact that all girls are romantic, and he should do everything in his power to keep alive the exaltation that comes to woman in love.

If, however, the girl finds herself engaged to a young man negligent in the details mentioned above, she should avoid rushing into an immediate marriage. Marrying to reform man of disagreeable habits, or to teach one's mate the common decencies or the ordinary manners and amenities of life usually ends as a nagging contest, developing in the victim a sense of social inferiority that is an endless source of unhappiness, and in the other the misery of paying an endless penalty for the mistake of an ill-advised marriage.

Most youths in the stage of development go through a series of awkward habits which are soon discarded. There are certain tendencies which are the result of early training and environment which may leave him, but which on the other hand may return when he is off guard or if he permits himself to sink into complacent self-sufficiency. It is a delicate problem to deal with. If the girl is clever she may cope with this and settle the problem once for all. But the first essential is to win the man's respect and confidence by the power of love, never to indulge in tactless and cruel destructive criticism. To help the young man in this fashion, through confidence and kindness, is often to prove that he has in truth chosen a real helpmate.

One indispensable truth the engaged girl must remember: The fiancé's breath, odor, touch, embrace and kiss must be pleasing to her. If they are not, if there is an impulsive or instinctive emotional and physical recoil, then under no circumstances should the engagement be prolonged. This requires courage and bravery. But do not forget that the life happiness of two persons is at stake.

The intimacies permitted during the engagement, the legitimate intimacies of kisses and caresses, in the protecting atmosphere of poetic romance, thus fulfil a distinct and all-important physiological function—the deepening of desire and the commingling of the spiritual and the physical. The engagement with its growing emotional bond is thus not merely a social convenience; it is the fulfillment of a necessary and vital process. The engagement continues the courting period. It is not the end of it. The bond should be tightened and strengthened, never loosened.

Lovemaking at this time becomes a tender and delicate process. The more exciting uncertainties have temporarily been settled. Responsibilities to one's self as well as to the loved one are increased. This is true particularly for the engaged girl. For while the lover may have too great a respect for the girl ever to reveal the depth and the power of his physical passion, her caresses may arouse him to a pitch beyond the power of his control. Young men have been known to seek relief through prostitutes or self-abuse. Here is another danger to be avoided. The girl who has attained a realization of her responsibilities must therefore aim always to keep uppermost

the spiritual aspect of the relation, so that
these trysts are a source of strength and courage and ambition to her fiancé instead of a
physical indulgence in excitements which cannot be satisfied.

By the spiritual aspect I do not mean sentimental rubbish. The engaged couple should
talk directly on matters bearing on their future
communal life and happiness; aims and am-
bitions; the possibility of having children.
They should read together—poetry, novels,
books which intensify their sense of the beauty
and the greatness of life. Frankness and honesty in matters of sex should not be avoided,
nor should the problem of modern marriage be
neglected. Both should aim to bring out of
the other latent ideas on all subjects.

The engaged girl owes it to herself to ascertain her fiancé's convictions concerning
marriage. Is he a prude or a hypocrite? Is
he woefully unconscious of his responsibilities?
Has he gained his knowledge of sex from experience, or from chance hearsay? Is his attitude toward women in general reassuring to
one who has selected him as her future husband? Is he willing to submit to a health
test?

I do not mean that the young woman should indulge in a legal cross-examination. But it is perfectly possible for her to find out on various opportunities answers to these questions, answers which may teach her much concerning the real nature of her fiancé. It is especially important to determine his attitude toward women in general. If it is gallant, chivalrous, generous and respectful, she may congratulate herself on her choice. If on the contrary, she discovers that his attitude is cynical, thoughtless, derogatory, domineering, or brutal, the girl may well break the engagement, no matter how enticing and tempting the man's offer may otherwise be. For sooner or later the girl who marries such a man may find herself the victim of this attitude.

With the greater independence which young women have acquired in this century, and the greater sense of equality, this type of man is gradually disappearing.

The question will inevitably be asked: How long should the engagement continue?

This is a question that depends upon individual circumstance and no general answer can be satisfactory. Nevertheless, there are certain general truths which appear self-evident.

I believe, first of all, that the day of the long engagement is past. Young people should marry, whenever that is possible, within a year after the announcement of the engagement. Unless one or the other is unavoidably separated, unless the case is exceptional, there is no good reason for a longer engagement.

Postponement is usually excused on the ground of financial inability. Experience and observation have shown me that the man who excuses himself as too poor to marry and who is waiting until he has enough, is either using this as an excuse or never does reach the point of solving his financial troubles.

A sound and happy marriage, with a young woman who is truly a helpmate and shares burdens equally, is the greatest aid to an ambitious young man. Instead of complicating them, marriage on this basis helps solve financial difficulties. No young man who is strong and ambitious should let poverty, real or supposed, stand in the way of marriage.

I do not advocate hasty, flighty, reckless marriages. Caution and prudence, on the other hand, can be carried to the point of disease, killing every fine impulse with delay and procrastination. It is possible to marry and live together on the same incomes necessary for the separate individuals, providing a family can be avoided for a few years.

The length of the engagement must be decided by the couple concerned. The culmination in marriage should be from the beginning its true objective.

The day of the wedding should be set far enough in advance to permit adequate preparations and plans for its successful outcome. For both there is excitement and nervous tension without adding the additional confusion of hurry and lack of preparation.

It is not always possible to set the exact day of the month, but the month may be chosen, and plans made for the general time.

It is advisable that the young woman should when possible set the day, taking care to avoid its coincidence with the menstrual period. Excitement, over-activity and overwork not infrequently bring about the menstrual flow several days before the regular and normal time. If for instance, this date is calculated to fall on May 5th-9th, it would be well to set the wedding day between the 15th and the 22nd of May, or any time of the intermenstrual period, except for one week before the next regular date.

If you are as "regular as clockwork," then you may accurately set the exact date. Eight to fourteen days after the beginning of the regular period would be the most advisable time. To spare the nerves and the constitution, it would be well for the bride-to-be to spend two days in bed at the time of the menstrual period. These two or three days of repose, away from noise and bustle, this respite from callers and telephone and undue excitement, will do much to restore poise and to regain the nervous energies often so carelessly expended in social activities during the final days of the engagement.

Peace and quiet are more essential to the happy fulfillment of this great event than the ceaseless round of social activities ordinarily indulged in. Absence from the fiancé at this period is also advisable. Such seclusion has a great psychological and physiological benefit that is never regretted. The girl is by this step enabled to return with strength and poise regained, her love rejuvenated and freshened.

She enters marriage with complete poise and strength, so that the wedding marks the beginning of her new life instead of entering matrimony fatigued, exhausted by excitement and nervous strain.

DEAR MRS. SANGER:

Knowing "open confession is good for the soul" I will go into this as fully yet as briefly as possible. During my two years of married life I detest and have a horror of natural sexual intercourse and have no desire or satisfaction even when I do cohabit with my husband. Naturally I have many times disappointed my husband and it causes little upsets and friction. I love him passionately and the present state of affairs cause me great mental suffering. Have had medical advice and treatment with no results; but have neglected owing to our doctor being a personal friend to tell him what I can tell you. Years ago when at a boarding school in England (my home) I with many others girls abused myself in many ways. This went on for many years as I was at that time very highly sexed. Am regular in my menstrual periods, fairly good health, except for high strung nerves, and slight hysterical attacks. Can you give me any advice as to whether the early abuse could be the cause of my present condition, and if it is an impossibility for me to return to normal? For my husbands sake wish to rectify this condition if it is possible and if you can give me any advice it would be more than appreciated.

MRS. G. A. F.

CHAPTER VI

THE HONEYMOON

THE importance of the first step into the conjugal life cannot be overemphasized. Initiation demands all the foresight, self-control and skill that the bridegroom can summon to his aid.

Before the advent of the single standard, this problem may not have been as complex as it is today. After the horrors of a bridal night, women have been known to leave inexperienced husbands forever.

For the bridegroom, therefore, the first essential is to realize and to dominate the whole situation. He seeks to escape from friends and relatives at the proper moment. He never loses sight of the primary and central importance of his behavior and his mastery of himself, always present is the aim to bring his marriage to a happy consummation.

Through inexperience, ignorance, and a lack of self-control, due to excitement, many bridegrooms have recklessly thrown away all possibilities of subsequent happiness. To avoid this, the wise husband seeks to understand more and more of the inner nature of the woman he is marrying.

The very young woman looks upon the wedding day in a very different light from the more mature woman. Until the age of twenty-three the young woman is most apt to be much less sophisticated and calmly philosophical than a more mature woman. To her the wedding day is all gaiety and romance. She has derived her idea of the nuptial festivities from novels or the motion pictures. Girls of this type are seldom satisfied with quiet weddings. She craves for excitement and hopes for all the picturesque and romantic features of the traditional wedding.

She knows only superficially the youth she is marrying. She knows that greater intimacies are to occur. She has heard older women friends, perhaps, discuss some aspects of marital relations. Perhaps her mother or an older married sister have given her some intimate advice and information: such information may be misinformation or misguiding. No one, at any rate, can teach her concerning her own private experiences and their psychological effect upon her. These things depend too much upon external conditions, upon the successful adjustment of feeling and emotion established by bride and groom.

No matter how much self-possession the girl may show outwardly, the approach of the wedding day fills her with a vague unconscious anxiety. The thrill of anticipation, of expected happiness, is not without an element of fear. She is taking a step into the unknown, venturing into an undiscovered country. Misgivings—Will her love be reciprocated after consummation?

Of small importance, in the conquest of happiness in marriage, are the outward festivities following the ceremony. Those are but accessories, the external trimmings which concern only the social relationship. Of infinitely greater importance are those hours when the bride and groom have at last attained privacy, when they find themselves "alone at last."

The custom of the wedding journey offers both advantages and disadvantages. Too often decisions concerning the bridal night are determined by train schedules and such exigencies. It should be obvious to all sensible people that a Pullman car is hardly suitable for the consummation of romance or a proper setting for the first conjugal embrace.

Hurry, bustle, and anxiety should be avoided. The change from the familiar home environment is not conducive to that sense of seclusion without which mutual enjoyment is rendered practically impossible. Nevertheless the confussion of travel, the embarrassment of finding oneself in the midst of strange faces, the impossibilities of sanitary and hygienic conveniences, the noise, the excitement and incidents of travel, all tend to increase the element of fear and morbid anxiety.

Such conditions are destructive to the proper consummation of marriage. Far more advisable is it to seek seclusion in a quiet hotel before undertaking any long railroad journey. In the event that this is impossible, the first conjugal embrace should be postponed until an atmosphere of peace and quiet is attained. Avoid hurry and confusion. Try to remember that your lifetime is ahead of you. A false step is worse than no step. Seek to discover the hidden traits in each other's nature. Recover from the nervous strain and excitement of the wedding festivities. There are secrets to be exchanged, confidences to be revealed, innocent pleasures in the novelty and the surprises of this new adventure to be enjoyed preceding the initiation.

The consummation of love cannot be brought as an incidental to the questionable pleasures of railroad travel, or sight-seeing and wandering about strange towns. Such pleasures bring with them actual physical fatigue as well as mental exhaustion occasioned by the never ceasing flood of new sights and sounds.

The burden of the engagement period has fallen upon the bride. The period of the honeymoon is essentially the responsibility of the bridegroom. Protective tenderness and delicacy and attention to his bride's emotional conditioin after her days and weeks of preparation and anticipation are imperative duties for him. He must remember that this is the culmination of the first period of her life. Long before she had even made his acquaintance, the girl has for years looked forward to this adventurous moment. No normal girl can be considered as not fearful of this novel and crucial experience. This change in her whole way of living has made the deepest impression upon her mind. To permit her to find herself to be mistress of her own emotions during this paramount psychic and physical experience, time, quiet, and rest are necessary.

Mainly through lack of adequate knowledge of the emotional nature of women, many impatient and selfish young husbands have plunged ahead to self-gratification with such reckless rapidity that the conjugal relation is forever afterwards associated in the woman's mind with a positive feeling of repulsion.

I realize that the mind of the young husband is also the battleground of conflicting ideas, emotions and instincts. For him also marriage is a new venture. He may be embarrassed, over-excited, a trifle oppressed by the sense of his great responsibility, perhaps a bit fearsome of his victory in his final ultimate conquest of the woman's heart.

Therefore he must make haste slowly. He must not forget that haste and hurry can defeat him more than deliberation and control. He cannot trust to blind instinct. He should previously seek definite and concrete scientific knowledge concerning the nature of physical love, knowledge not merely of the sexual function of the generative organs of the male, but of the female as well, and their relation to the psychic constitution of both sexes. By such enlightenment the young bride will also be spared an untold amount of unnecessary suffering. Both bride and groom will understand that the perfect and desirable consummation of love is the outcome of mutual respect and consideration and that, in many cases, this adjustment is not attained immediately but sometimes after days and weeks. Both must learn to look upon their bodies and the organs of sex as delicate instruments for the expression of love. They must patiently learn the rudiments of the art of love before attaining perfection.

The first approach by the bridegroom is a step of the utmost importance. It makes the deepest and often a life-long impression upon the memory of the woman.

Too many men assume a matter-of-fact attitude, and take everything for granted. Aiming perhaps to exhibit complete mastery of the situation, they proceed as if the whole matter were a casual act, the perfunctory right of the marriage ceremony. Others, themselves embarrassed, mistakenly try to make light of the situation, or conceal their own lack of knowledge by assuming the mask of superiority, the "know-it-all" attitude.

Combined with a careless conduct, painful to the young wife during the honeymoon, such an attitude has been known to poison from its beginning the course of married life, and has been the ultimate cause of separation. It is imperative that the husband confine his attentions to the bride, and not exhibit interest in other women. Nothing can be more humiliating to a bride than to be forced to realize that she is not the center of her husband's attention, supreme in his interest.

The memory of her husband's ill-concealed admiration for other women, their looks, their clothes, their various attractions—rankled in the heart of one bride throughout her married life of twenty years until divorce became the only solution. She told me of the undying memory of that unhappy honeymoon, when bitter jealousy was born in her heart; the maladjustment, the petty quarreling and the growing bitterness became with the passing of the years bitterly intolerable. In this case the husband may have been technically innocent. But he was a clumsy wooer, and began his marriage with a fatal mistake.

Another young husband found his life turned topsy-turvy the day following his brilliant and gorgeous wedding. His bride was a cheerful, radiantly happy girl who had looked forward to marriage with the man she loved as the culmination of happiness.

This man took his bride to a hotel where a luxurious suite had been reserved for them. As he had done everything possible to make his bride happy, he was amazed, in waking up the following morning to find his young wife sitting up in a chair. She was sobbing as though her heart had been broken. Try as he could, he was unable to discover the source of her secret sorrow. Weeks passed into months. Outwardly the young wife appeared contented. Nevertheless she gradually grew pale and nervous, until finally her doctor prescribed a rest cure.

A long time afterwards this wife confided to a friend that she had suffered a terrific shock of disappointment on her bridal night. During courtship, her fiancé's advances had been sufficient to arouse her expectations to the highest point. On the wedding night his approach and embraces had been in the order of a hurried meal over a lunch counter. This duty perfunctorily performed, the young husband, quite oblivious to his bride's sharp disappointment, had promptly fallen into a deep slumber.

Astounded at his lack of idealism, and crushed by the total collapse of her romance, this young bride lay awake throughout the long night, thinking of all she had expected, of the long weeks of preparation, of her wedding garments unnoticed, and her husband's bland indifference to all of her attractive preparations. Tears had finally been her only relief. And so the conviction took root in her mind, a conviction that became ineradicable, that the whole meaning of marriage was to men to be found in the attitude of her husband. That all he wanted was perfunctory sex gratification. For her, irretrievably, the beauty, the poetry, the exaltation of romance had been dragged in the dust and had come to an end.

The most successful bridegroom is he who approaches this act of communion and consummation in a spirit of reverence. The awe and the mystery of this remarkable gift so profoundly impresses the young man standing thus on the threshold of life that his approach is but the outward expression of his declaration of love, of adoration, of worship. Here is the time when as never before the young husband should establish the confidence of his wife in the physical and spiritual unity of his love.

He must never forget that this is the initiation of his beloved. The atmosphere, the surroundings, every detail is of the utmost importance. Unimportant as they may seem to the young man, women often carry through life these things as indelible memories. Women have been known to cling to men through poverty, sickness, destitution, even of cruelty to themselves and their children, because of such treasured memories, of promises made and consideration shown, and the undying freshness of the recollection of the first embrace which consecrated her love.

Many of the mistakes and missteps made by young husbands are the outcome of inexperience and embarrassment. But ignorance is no longer a valid excuse. It is the duty of every young man entering matrimony to forearm himself with authentic knowledge. While the family physician is adequate to consult in matters concerning his own male organization, and even of the physical function, he needs more knowledge than that. Nowadays it is possible to talk frankly with some women older and more experienced in life. The advice needed for a successful wedding journey and honeymoon would willingly be given by an older woman or man—preferably not a member of one's own family—and a thorough understanding obtained of the bridegroom's duties.

INITIATION FOR THE BRIDE

The bride should likewise make adequate preparation for the first physical embrace. Modesty and delicacy have their rightful place here as in all phases of life, but modesty and purity do not mean prudishness and false reticence. There is a time and place for all things. Young brides in entering this most sacred of human relations should not hamper themselves by false notions of propriety.

The girl who is too prudish to make preparations beforehand for the event which she knows is bound to take place is most likely to fail to establish a human and happy relationship with her young husband. Often such brides become immediately pregnant. Before they have experienced marital love they are on the way to premature motherhood. Moreover, her hampering inhibitions may erect a barrier between her real desires and the possibility of realizing them. Until she casts them aside, liberates herself, she cannot experience the deepest love for her mate.

The sensible girl entering marriage will have forearmed herself with definite knowledge, both of her own nature, and that of the man she has chosen as a life companion. Especially will she seek to understand and to recognize the overpowering urgent passion of her beloved at the first consummation of their marriage.

No precise rules and regulations can here be advised for conduct during the first fortnight. At best the honeymoon is an abnormal period. Emotions are heightened. Each experience is a new adventure. Often the effort of mutual adjustment is a slow process. The bride must be lenient and sympathetic to the young husband. She should try to understand and help him.

Among some women the membrane known as the hymen, which partially closes the entrance to the vagina is very tough. Among others it is scarcely perceptive or even totally absent. Its presence or absence indicates nothing. The virgin may be without this particular membrane, may not have been born with one, while many married women may still possess the hymen intact. Therefore its absence should occasion no worry to the wife-to-be. The old superstition that the intact hymen indicated virginity is no longer accepted by informed people.

It may be found, however, that complete consummation cannot take place for several days because of the resistance of this membrane. Or its rupture may cause severe pain. In this case patience must be cheerfully used by both mates. The pain will soon be overcome.

Aside from the caresses and intimacies of her beloved, it is not unusual for the bride to find at first no particular physical delight in the sexual embrace. This lack of pleasure is also only temporary. By considerate effort and proper guidance and understanding any normal woman may be enabled to share with her husband the fullest joy in sex communion.

Among the essential preparations toward this end she should obtain advice concerning the hygienic accessories quite as necessary to her happiness as attractive clothing.

Sane and frank discussion of sexual relations between the young husband and wife is emphatically recommended. Such discussion facilitates mutual understanding and adjustment and does a great deal toward the solution of intimate problems. If possible the young couple should equip themselves with a reliable book or two by dependable authorities in which such problems are elucidated. This will bring them both to the realization that their case is not exceptional but that all newly married couples have the same road to travel, the same problem of establishing sexual harmony, the same great adventure of initiation into life.

No less than her husband, the young woman who values her future and who realizes that married happiness cannot be won except through effort, mutual understanding and adjustment, will look at the central truths of human life squarely and reliantly. Intelligently will she weave this beautiful but difficult thread into the fabric of her life and create out of it the pattern of married happiness.

Ultimately, despite the difficulties of initiation she must dominate the relation. This she knows vaguely even unconsciously: she must create the happiness of their life together. The future depends on the woman's attitude toward sex. If that attitude be one of fear, of shame, of anxiety, of ignorance masking itself in the guise of simpering innocence, (an attitude popularized in the Victorian novels of the last century) then only the redoubled efforts of the husband may save that marriage from failure.

If the bride brings to her marriage the antiquated attitude that sex expression is lustful, bestial, only a necessary concession to the animal impulse of the male, while she herself is spiritually superior to sex impulse, then indeed, her marriage is foredoomed to failure.

If on the other hand, the bride brings intelligence as well as a warmly pulsating personality to this relation, if she realizes that sex and all its functions are a necessary and even the most beautiful part of life and of happiness in marriage,—such a woman enters marriage with a certainty of winning joy and of developing all of its latent possibilities for a full and fruitful life. She enters marriage knowing that it is in human experience the greatest of all adventures. And in this adventure the woman will realize that she is the leader, the commander. She will realize that her weapons in crossing this unexplored, undiscovered country must be patience, tenderness understanding and knowledge and with these a challenging determination to wrest from marriage all of the happiness that rightfully belongs to her.

Her successful initiation into the joys of sexual love will destroy old prejudices, immature limitations, false and superficial values. The young wife will awaken to the direct and immediate application to herself of that profound truth of the poet who exclaimed:

> "Be not ashamed, women, your privilege encloses the rest, and is the exit of the rest.
> You are the gates of the body, and you are the gates of the soul."

DEAR MRS. SANGER:

I do not know if you are the right person to understand me or not but hope so. My husband is 23 and old for his age. I am 30 and considered by every one young for my age, so I cannot think that would make any difference in our love for each other. We have been married about 2½ years and we have the dearest boy any one ever was blessed with, 14 months old. I can hardly understand how we ever got him though. Although very fond of children I am so against sexual relations that I really feel insulted if my husband mentions anything about such things. I love my husband dearly but it seems I cannot love him in that way. He calls it love, I call it torture. I always had the idea that there should only be intercourse when children are desired, and I cannot have any more. I had such a time with this one. I was in bed ten weeks and the doctor didn't think I would ever get up. So I know that I must not. I would go through it again or even death before I would take a little life after it was started for I believe it murder.

My husband has left me four times and always says it is because I can't love him in that way, but it seems I just can't. He is very affectionate and good to me when we are together. I want to do what is right, what God would have us do. But I do not know what it is and I want a happy home so badly that is why I am appealing to you for help if there is any. If you have time I would appreciate a personal letter from you and any suggestions that you make I will try and follow. Is there any thing to be done in our case. So that my husband would not care for me in that way, or if it is right that we should, or is there any way that I could learn to care for him.

MRS. K. R.

CHAPTER VII

THE ORGANS OF SEX AND THEIR FUNCTIONS

"If anything is sacred, the human body is sacred,
  And the glory and sweet of a man, is the token of
    manhood untainted;
  And in man and woman, a clean, strong well-fibred
    body is beautiful as the most beautiful face."
                                        —*Whitman.*

NO young man or woman should marry
    without first securing a scientific under-
standing of the anatomy and functions of both
male and female organs of generations. This
understanding is essential to health and married happiness.

The sex organs are the instruments of love
expression. Upon their health depends the
entire health of body and mind. They are intimately connected, physiologically and psychologically with the nerves and glands in
every part of the body.

In every gesture, in the carriage, the voice,
the complexion, the depth and brightness of

the eyes, and in innumerable other ways, men and women reveal their happiness or unhappiness, their general tone and radiance of sex health or lack of it.

The sex organs are delicately organized instruments intimately and intricately related to all the avenues of the senses by which the mind is stimulated. The generative organs are in close relation with the central nervous system, interacting through this system, responding to impulses, desires and inhibitions, exerting a profound and immediate influence upon the emotional and physiological life.

These organs are also the glands of internal secretion, a part of the glandular system of the body. The great importance of this system is the latest great discovery of medical science. Secretions released and sent directly into the blood stream by the sex glands, as by other glands of the same system, are known as *hormones* or chemical messengers, almost too minute to be studied by the microscope, yet of the utmost importance in the building up and sustaining of bodily health.

The various hormones released by the different ductless glands, working together, are determining agents in building up health. If their action is unbalanced, if these hormones are in conflict, ill health results.

Therefore, the sex organs are not things apart. Their importance can no longer be neglected. Intelligent men and women now recognize the necessity of knowing themselves thoroughly. They must courageously insist on understanding all the vital functions of their bodies.

Let me again remind the youth and maid that in approaching marriage, they must not permit prudishness or a false sense of delicacy to stand in the way of acquiring this invaluable knowledge, not merely of the sex organs of their own sex, but of the opposite as well.

The successful consummation of marriage depends upon the adjustment of these organs, the interrelation and the harmonious interplay of the organs of generation. Without this mutual adjustment an abundant love-life is rendered impossible, for it is through these instruments that the emotion of love between husband and wife finds complete and culminating expression.

Let us briefly consider these instruments of the body. The first great and striking difference between the male and female organs of generation is to be found in the fact that the male organs are for the most part external organs, while the female are internal. The testicles of the man, two in number, are in a pouch or sack called the scrotum. This bag is composed of very thin skin containing no fat, which shrinks when exposed to cold and relaxes in condition of fatigue or extreme warmth. Usually the left testicle is slightly larger than the right, and the left half of the scrotum hangs lower. The testicles are semi-hard ovoid glands, made up of great quantities of fine tubes grouped in lobes or lobules. The products of the testicles are the life-giving sperm cells (spermatozoa) and the secretion or *hormone* known as the *gonad,* that glandular secretion which released directly into the blood stream confers manhood and masculine virility to the individual. Voronoff claims these *hormones* secreted by the testicles to be a veritable elixir of life. They are released throughout the entire period of sexual maturity, and are increasingly stimulated by a full and healthy abundant love-life.

The *vas deferens* is the duct or tube that carries away the sperm cells from the testicle (or testes) to store them inside the body in the seminal vesicles. These latter are reservoirs—which are nothing more than large irregular dilatations of the tubes themselves and are found lying behind and under the bladder, in front of the rectum.

The prostate gland, one of the most important organs of the male generative structure, is made up of three lobes. It is adjacent to the vesicles and the urethral canal passes through this gland as it passes from the bladder.

Under the stimulation of sexual excitement the penis, which is the intromittent organ of the male, becomes rigid. This condition is brought about by the swelling and fillting (or turgescence) of the three bundles of erectile tissue which compose this organ. Two bundles—known as the *corpora cavernosa*—are bodies of hollows or cells—begin on the under side of the pelvic bone and end in the glans penis, or head of the organ. A third or spongy body encloses the urethra, the canal through which both the urine is emitted and the semen ejaculated. This process is controlled by nerves, through which the erotic impulses from the brain are sent, and are located in the lumbar or lower part of the spinal cord.

The penis is enveloped by a thin skin, which

unless circumcision has been performed, protects the head or glans penis. This protective integument is known as the foreskin or prepuce. The head or corona of the penis is the most highly sensitive part of that organ. Numerous small glands near the free margin of the foreskin emit a secretion. Cleanliness to prevent irritation to this sensitive part should be taught from childhood. The necessity for such cleanliness was early recognized by certain tribes—notably the Jews—in establishing the practice of circumcision, cutting off the foreskin in early infancy. Today this custom is approved for reasons of hygiene.

Erection of the penis is occasioned by the dilatation of its blood vessels. First of all the bulbous or proximal part of the organs increases in size. The swelling extends through the two cavernous bodies and in a short time reaches the head or glans. The veins of the penis are said to be traversed by five times as much blood during erection as when in repose. This increase in the amount of blood is accompanied by a corresponding rise in temperature of the parts.

It should be evident that this sexual apparatus, in its mechanisms, its nervous organization, its glandular importance, is very sensitively organized. To control and direct the coursing impulses and emotions which come under sexual stimulus is a difficult art, yet it must be mastered by the young husband who wishes above all else to achieve happiness for the woman he loves and thus for himself.

The sex organs of the woman are as we have stated mostly internal, as contrasted with those of the male. Yet there are striking similarities, or rather analogous and complementary aspects. Thus the two ovaries correspond to the testicles of the male; like the testicles they secrete hormones of the utmost importance to the well-being and general health of the woman.

The other organs—the vulva, clitoris, and vagina—likewise correspond in certain aspects and are skillfully constructed for mutual adjustment in the symphony of love.

Vagina means sheath or scabbard. It is made up of this muscular tissue and mucous membrane. Ordinarily collapsed the vagina is capable of enormous expansion, as it becomes the canal through which the child passes at birth. The tissue of the vagina is wrinkled and corrugated. It is furnished with glands which at the time of sexual excitement secrete a lubricating fluid essential in copulation.

In the folds and wrinkles of the vagina may be hidden the sperm cells deposited by the penis. The male sperm may live there for several days unless sterilized.

The length of the vagina varies in women. As in the case of the male penis, it is not necessarily small in small bodies, nor large in large women. As its walls are composed of erectile tissue it is always capable of expansion to adjust itself to the need.

At the front of the vulva is found the clitoris, the special seat of sex sensitiveness in woman. Like the penis in the male this diminutive organ contains numerous sensory nerve endings. It is highly sensitive during copulation.

The womb, or uterus, lies between the bladder and the rectum, and is one of the most important of the generative organs in the female. In shape the womb is like a pear hanging with the stem downward. The small end or neck is known as the cervix. The uterus is set down in the vagina much as an egg rests in an egg cup. During consummation the womb, which may be described as a muscular organ, undergoes a series of peristaltic compressions and contractions by means of which the ejaculated semen may be drawn into its hollow cavity. The womb becomes for nine months the "nest" of the conceived child. The muscles of the uterus expand continuously until the time of birth, when the infant passes through the vaginal canal out of the body.

The womb is suspended by muscles in the pelvic region. It is elastic as well as tough in its own muscular envelope. But when its muscular action is weakened, this organ falls down into the vaginal canal. This condition is often responsible for the pain occasioned to some women at the time of intercourse.

The upper part of the womb is connected with the Fallopian tubes, which correspond with the vas deferens in the male. The Fallopian tubes connect the uterus, or womb, with the two ovaries. They are serpentine in shape and it is through these tubes that the ova or egg cells come into the womb where they await development after conception has taken place. The ova (eggs) are discharged from the ovary at the time of menstruation—usually every twenty-eight days for normal women.

The ovaries, which correspond somewhat to the male testicles, are two almond-shaped organs lying on each side of the uterus. It is in the ovaries that the female cells are grown. But in contrast to the male cells which are ejaculated through the urethra either during intercourse or by nocturnal emission, the ova are deposited in the uterus and discharged each month if not fertilized by the sperm cell.

The hymen (or "maidenhead") is a thin membrane which, if present, partly closes the vaginal canal. Sometimes this membrane completely surrounds the opening, sometimes it is crescent shaped. Its presence was once thought a symbol of virginity, but accidents in childhood may cause its rupture, or it may never have been formed. Its absence should never be considered as indicating a previous sex relation in an unmarried woman.

Intimately connected with the genital organs of the female and to a large extent influenced by the glandular secretions from the ovaries are the breasts, secondary features of great importance, both sexually and from their functions in motherhood. During puberty the breasts of the girl develop considerably. With many women the breast enlarges during the period of menstruation, thus indicating their organic relation with the function of the ovaries and the womb. The skin above the nipple is very delicate, of a pinkish color in women before children are born and darker after.

The breasts are considered an integral feature of feminine beauty. They are moreover important and highly sensitive centers of stimulation.

Dear Madam:—

I will take the liberty to write you a few lines and hope you will not think I am bold as I have heard a lot about you where you have helped others and hope you can help me.

I am a young man of 35 and married and for the past year I have been little or nothing to my wife in regards to sexual relations and cannot understand the cause as I am not one that has abused myself.

I have tried to keep this secret from my wife all this time as I dont know how she will take it, I have told her that my work is a little heavy and I am a little run down but thats a lie as my work isn't any harder today than it was five years ago.

I have taken treatments from a physician for the last six months but no results.

Last spring I obtained for my wife one of your books "The women and the New Race" and she has found it a great little helper so I am taking this course with the hopes that you will be in a position to know of some remedy that will be of help to me.

Thanking you in advance for your trouble and very sorry if I have done any wrong in writing to you about my case.

I remain

C. P.

CHAPTER VIII

THE DRAMA OF LOVE—THE PRELUDE

"I would like to suggest, with great respect, that an addition be made to the objects of marriage in the Marriage Service, in these terms: 'The complete realisation of the love of this man and this woman, the one for the other.'"

—*Lord Dawson of Penn, at the Church Congress, Birmingham, England, 1921.*

THERE is no greater need, at the present time, than a frank, serious and reverential education of men and women in the innermost problems of the marriage relation.

Upon the complete realization of the love of husband for wife and wife for husband depends not only the enduring happiness of marriage, but also, to a far greater extent than most people realize, success in life and the release and direction of those hidden vital energies that are so essential to the peace and security which create those values so essential for creature living.

If, on the other hand, the love expression be

frustrated, disappointment and disillusion and discord usurp the place of joy and contentment; then harmonious adjustment of the two individuals is rendered tragically impossible. These are the factors which destroy marriage, and which lead often to the divorce court.

When we consider the woeful tragedies of wrecked lives, the silent suffering and the wasteful sacrifice of joy and human energy which have for countless generations been brought about by leaving this, the most important function of human life, to chance and ignorance, we cannot escape the conclusion that the cost of silence is too high, and that it is high time for husbands and wives—particularly those who stand at the threshold of life —to approach the intricate problems of the love-relation with the same intelligence and insight and understanding of human nature required for success in other spheres of human endeavor.

The present chapters are written in a spirit of profound reverence, in the hope that they may help those young men and women who stand at the entrance of life's labyrinth to avoid the pitfalls and disasters that have been

occasioned in the past by those unfortunate
humans who did not dare tear asunder the thin
cobweb veil of prudishness and misunderstanding
and whose precious lives have been wrecked
because, while standing so near to marital happiness, they failed to attain that mutual adjustment which should have been the most
priceless treasure of their lives.

At the very outset, let us frankly confess
that the problems of mutual adjustment of two
persons in the love relationship cannot be
solved by the mere reading of a book, or a
slavish dependence upon "directions." Each
marriage is an individual problem, to be solved
only by the participants. Happiness in marriage does not spring full grown from the
bridal bed. To endure, it must be won gradually. It is like a tree; it must first plant its
roots in a fertile nourishing soil. It must be
carefully nurtured, cared for, studied and directed. Once firmly rooted, drawing nourishment from the rich soil of mutual joy and deepening harmony, it grows steadily and strongly,
and in its turn returns tenfold to those who
have tended it the joy and happiness it represents. I would even go so far as to state that
there is no other source of true contentment

or understanding of life values than that which comes from the realization of love in marriage.

There are, however, certain primary considerations of the utmost importance which are indispensable in guiding the young husband away from those missteps and pitfalls and ill-timed actions which have in the past often proved permanently disastrous to the marriage relation.

He must at all times remember that he must be careful not to shock or injure the delicate nervous system of his beloved and for this reason must adequately prepare her for the consummation of their love.

To be the master of his passion instead of its slave is the first essential rule in love etiquette every young husband must learn.

He must learn to control the tumultuous power of his impulses. Through each act of the great love drama he must learn to direct this great power which wells up within his own nature. Unaware of the force of the desire that is released in the excitement of this new experience, too many young men have succumbed to the temptation of casting discretion to the winds and permitting passion to find unchecked expression. Such behavior is essentially selfish; and selfishness in the love-relation is fatal to true happiness.

The successful husband-lover will, during every act of the love drama, seek to redirect all egotistical impulses, and, like a skillful driver, at every moment hold himself under intelligent control.

He is enabled to accomplish this seemingly difficult feat by concentrating his attention not upon his own heightening desire, but upon that of his beloved. He will be helped in the accomplishment of this highly desirable end if he can bring himself to observe a few simple rules of conduct which will heighten to an unsuspected degree the joy of his partner and will thus repay him by increasing his skill as a lover. These rules are:

1. *Avoid hurry.* Only on the firm foundation of adequate preparation may the consummation of the love act be satisfactorily fulfilled for both participants. Time is an essential ingredient to successful love making.

2. *Avoid violence.* Remember that true strength may and should express itself gently. It is the man who is not confident of his own strength who seeks to reassure himself by violent and abrupt actions. The successful hus-

band realizes that his beloved is a delicately organized nature, and he refrains from seeking to impose his desire prematurely upon her. Instead he aims to awake her love nature to the point at which she will express her desire for consummation.

3. Seek first of all to allay nervous fears and apprehension. An atmosphere of complete peace and confidence is essential to the culmination of the love-relation. Sex communion gains measurably by careful preparation and a slow and retarded progress through the all-important stage of preparation.

Without the harmony of the prelude, the flight into spiritual ecstasy cannot be accomplished.

Remember that sex communion is not to be regarded as a single act, but is composed of several essential parts, or acts as in a drama.

As in a musical symphony, each part is distinct in its movement and progress, leading without break into the succeeding action. In the technique of love, which is mastered gradually by intelligent and unselfish guidance, each part of this drama requires adequate fulfillment. Each stage unfolds to the participants its own delight and intensifies the joy revealed by each succeeding link in the chain of this creative experience.

Physiologically and emotionally the male is so constituted that, once stimulated, he finds himself almost immediately prepared for action. Psychologically, therefore, he is apt to neglect the task of preparing his beloved for their mutual flight together to the high realm of ecstasy. But if this flight is to be a triumphant one, his first duty is to awake her desire for this flight. He must awaken her senses and her soul. He must arouse that indefinable something in her which makes her his best beloved.

He alone can accomplish this. For the desire of the wife can be awakened by her loved one only. By his caresses, which may be likened to the gentle touches of a composer whose fingers begin an improvisation on the keyboard of his piano, by his revelation of his understanding of her emotional life, his knowledge of her deeper nature, he may arouse her latent or sleeping desire. Once he has inspired her confidence he may discover by her response the proper moment for proceeding to the next link in the chain of ecstasy. Because he focusses his attention upon the desire of his beloved, aiming always to heighten it and intensify it, the young husband is all the better able to control his own surging passion. At all times he is gentle; but with an aggressive gentleness, realizing that in the initial stages his is the active yet controlled part.

His first duty is the preparation of the hidden, deepest nature of his beloved to receive his love. In opening the portals of her being, or better still in persuading the woman to open these secret portals and to receive him, the young husband deepens and intensifies tenfold the love nature of his partner. In leading her successfully, nay triumphantly, through this mysterious initiation he becomes for her a veritable god—worthy of her profoundest worship. He is sharing with her the greatest and most unforgettable adventure of her life. This experience is the true marriage, the weaving of ties of ecstasy that bind, ties of fidelity and loyalty.

Once he realizes that the whole foundation of martial happiness—and with this a large part of his own spiritual and material well-being—is intricately bound up with his behavior and habits in the most intimate experience of life, the young husband will not be so foolish as to risk leaving this delicate problem to chance. He will prepare himself by seeking the counsel of older and wiser men and discuss with them in a serious and reverent vein the problems of initiation.

First of all he must learn that the sexual nature of man differs profoundly from that of woman. Under stimulation the sexual nature of man asserts itself almost instantaneously ready for action. Due to tradition and by nature, physiologically as well as psychologically, the sex nature of woman is more deeply hidden in the mysterious recesses of her being. More deeply concealed, it is not so immediately susceptible to stimulation, is far slower in response and thus is not immediately ready for the act of love.

In addition to these considerations, women are less apt, by education and training, by tradition and repressions induced by early education, to associate the idea of love with its direct bodily expression. Fortunately the era of prudishness is now passing. But even though the bride approaches the initiation with modest frankness, the bridegroom should never forget that the average woman of normal health and vigor requires at least twenty minutes to a half hour for the completion of the act of preparation alone.

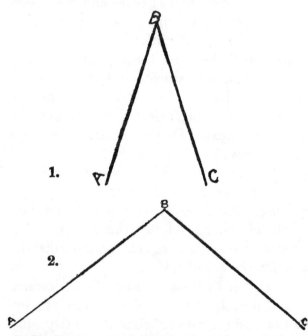

1. The line from *a* to *b* indicates the quick ascent of sexual desire in man.

2. The same line indicates the less rapid ascent of desire in woman.

To hurry through this essential stage is fatal to the successful fulfillment of all that follows. Hurry and violence are conducive to undue excitement and nervousness, of tightening tension instead of relaxation and confidence, which are essential to securing the rhythmic sense of freedom in action.

The young husband therefore aims to attune her mind no less than her body for the harmonic consummation of love. He seeks to remove all obstacles from the path of their triumphant love flights—the petty obstacles of worries, fears, inhibitions, all signs of fatigue or external influences that might invade the peace of mind and break the chain of ardor and desire in its successive links.

There is, as an example, the delicate problem of the lighting in the room. Shall this mysterious rite be acted in total darkness or in a delicate semi-obscurity. Certainly illumination has much to do with the creation of a mood. This is merely one of the minor problems for the husband—he must find out his wife's preference. Most women undoubtedly prefer to blot out from their consciousness all reminders of time and place; though here as in all such questions, tastes vary, and the chivalrous husband will undertake to fulfill the slightest wishes of his wife in all such matters, no matter how whimsical or unreasoning they may strike him.

The ancient story of Pygmalion and Gala-
tea contains a valuable symbolic lesson for the
most modern of young husbands. Like Pygmalion's, his task is to bring to life the real
woman of flesh and blood concealed in the
statue he adores. It is the duty of the lover
to accomplish this miracle by using all the resources he has at his command, and with a
technique as skillful as that of any sculptor.
He aims to wipe from her consciousness any
misgivings concerning defects, and to emphasize her loveliness. He removes her shyness
and embarrassment by repeating over and over
again in whispered terms of endearment his
admiration and worship of her loveliness.
Step by step, ever so gently, he leads her into
a mysterious realm of enchantment, of poetry
and adoration.

She will find herself no longer a mere girl
of flesh and blood, a wild duckling or Cinderella, but in every truth a fairy princess. At
this point, it is imperative that the young husband concentrate upon the psychic condition
and mood of his beloved. He must note her
response to his caresses, the caresses of a true
artist, of a Pygmalion who begins to feel the

flesh and blood course and pulsate under the influence of his gentle touch.

He must ascertain if her response denotes the awakening of real passion, or whether this response remains merely childishly affectionate.

Has passion, the passionate love of the mature woman begun now to well out from the fathomless well of her deepest nature in response to his own surging desire? This question must be answered before the act of preparation is successfully completed. The answer must be: Yes.

The caresses of the young bridegroom must be at all times gentle and yet stimulating, and have a definite aim and direction. The skillful lover is especially careful at every point of this progress to avoid any act or gesture which might tend to destroy or flatten out (as a musical note sung out of key) the rising tide of his beloved's desire.

Physiologically the effect of this prelude is to stimulate the nerve-endings of the vagina and vulva, and to release those mysterious lubricating secretions which indicate the preparedness of the special organs for the act of communion in love.

For the young girl who is thus initiated into womanhood, it is necessary to bring to this new experience dignity and honesty. She will cast aside the unthinking silliness and levity of girlhood as she must cast aside the hindering garments and fashions of the outer world. She must remember that hers is to be no mere passive part in the final enactment of the love drama, and that its beauty and passionate poetry must not be marred by the discordant note of false prudishness, for in the terms of the Bible, husband and wife are no longer twain but one flesh.

She must learn to give, to give freely, to give completely. And this generous gesture,—the gesture of a Greek goddess in its grave, solemn joy,—can only be worthy of her love when it is enacted with those large ample movements suggestive of relaxation and peace.

She must learn therefore to relax. She must seek to fall into the rhythm of the love flight, as the continuation of a dance, a dance of soul as well as body, a dance in which two humans are not longer separate and distinct persons, but in which their beings are co-mingled in a new and higher unity.

Nor should it be forgotten, in this matter

of prelude or preparation for sex communion, that all the everyday relations between husband and wife in reality constitute the prelude for the ritual of sexual communion. They are likewise also indications of the success or failure in the attainment of mutual ecstasy. Each thoughtful act, each gesture of love and consideration, is likely to have a cumulative effect adding to and enhancing the celebration of sex communion, and deepening the enduring love between husband and wife.

And on the other hand, petty disagreements and unkind words are often deplorable indications of the failure of husband and wife to attain that mutual rhythm and ecstasy which is so essential to happiness in marriage.

DEAR MRS. SANGER:

Can you tell me why I am incapable of any feeling whatever during "family relation" with my husband, and if the condition can be corrected in any way. I want to live up to my part of the bargain in building up a happy home, but it cant be done on pretense, and no man who is impulsive and affectionate wants a wife who is cold and reserved. I love my husband very much, he is thoughtful and affectionate, but living with him as his wife gives me no pleasure. Can it be that outside interests, or some condition of my health could cause this? I am, apparently, in excellent health and have a young son six months old, and have enjoyed the best of health before and after his birth, which was perfectly normal in every way. If you can suggest something that will be of benefit to me, I will certainly appreciate it.

MRS. N. R. F.

CHAPTER IX

SEX COMMUNION—THE FULFILMENT

"They are no more twain,—but one flesh."
—*Matthew xix.6.*

WE have seen the necessity for a prolonged and definite period of preparation. This preparation is directed toward the accomplishment of certain definite ends. It is not merely waiting or aimless delay. One of its most valuable fruits is in training the impatient husband to retain control and guidance over his rebellious impulses. By exercising his skill as a lover, he succeeds in awakening in his wife true, legitimate passion, instead of inducing her merely to submit as a passive partner to the love-embrace. In the one case she is an active and equal partner; in the second, marriage is merely a cloak covering an act of seduction—or even of spiritual rapine.

In the second stage, by which the spiritual union of man and wife is given definite physical and bodily expression, there must likewise be no reckless abandon to hurried brutality. It should not be forgotten that this union is most effective and harmonious when there is no constraint of movement and both husband and wife are free to express the ecstasy of communion.

At the completion of the physical union of body and spirit, it is highly desirable that the participants strain the impulse to abandon control and to plunge forward into a precipitate movement toward the climax. This is a temptation that should at all costs be avoided.

At this point, it is again necessary to consider the love-flight in the terms of music. The first definite climax has been attained. The crest of the first rhythmic wave has been reached. In order that the subsequent rhythm may reach an even higher crest, there must now follow a momentary ebb, after which mutual passion and ecstasy are permitted to surge again to greater heights and to produce even more exquisite thrills of ecstasy and joy.

Therefore, follows a brief moment of rest, a period which permits the husband to regain the control, that might at this point escape even the strongest-willed of men. It is for the young wife a moment which definitely focusses her awakened passion and permits her to prepare herself for the culminating flight which follows. In order that the rhythmic movements of the participants may not be impeded, mutual adjustments may be necessary.

At this point above all others, it is imperative that the husband shall not succumb to the temptation of merely satisfying his own bodily need. In the profoundest sense of the word, he must husband his resources and aim to bring to a climactic expression his wife's deepest love.

Thus, while it is imperative that the woman should release her own deep impulses and give them full and unashamed expression, it is essential that the husband, with a deep effort of the subconscious will, attune his own desire to hers and aim to reach a climax simultaneously with that of his beloved. In the ordinary normal woman this may be more retarded than the man might expect, gauging her nature by his own.

Here is the crux of the marital problem. For centuries women have been taught by custom and prejudice, especially in countries in which the Puritanic tradition dominates, that hers should be a passive, dutiful rôle—to sub-

mit but not to participate. Likewise men have
been schooled by tradition to seek mere selfish
gratification. This lack of constructive experience is responsible for the thousands of
unhappy marriages and the tragic wasted lives
of many wives, cheated by thoughtlessness and
ignorance of their legitimate right to marital
joy.

Much would be accomplished if women were
taught to be active, and men to check the
tumultuous expression of their passion.

Therefore, having attained legitimate freedom of expression, the wife will recognize that
she has an active part to play. She is now
fully aroused. She does not seek to suppress
or control her emotions at all. She must not
seek to crush down the passion which wells
up from her deepest nature. On the contrary:
she should and must abandon herself to it
utterly.

Dominated by erroneous ideas of propriety
and modesty, many women have in this experience failed to attain that joyful ecstasy
which is the legitimate fruit of marriage. The
true wife will not be ashamed to give expression to her passionate love for her husband.
For in so doing, she may be assured that he

will be proud of the passion he has brought to life within her nature and that its full-flowered expression will intensify and increase his love manifold. Its benefits will be reciprocal.

A preliminary failure does not mean that success may not be eventually attained. And when this triumph over difficulties is finally attained, mutual happiness will be all the greater. The love of husband for wife and wife for husband can find no more beautiful expression than in this mutual effort to create for the beloved the joy one hopes to experience in the love embrace. This joy is the finest flower of monogamy; and the miracle of undying love is the fruit of such experience.

The husband should aim to control his emotions. Rather than to permit purely physical impulses to dominate, he may master the strong current of passion that is coursing through his body by dwelling on the inner harmony, the spiritual mystery of this communion of two natures and the poetry of the experience. If the purely physical aspect threatens to usurp command, the heightened, accelerated rhythm may be brought for a few necessary moments to a standstill, while words of love, tenderness and reverence are whispered to the beloved. The effect will be magical.

Experience will teach the husband to watch for and to recognize in his beloved the approach of the culminating ecstasy. Not until this point is attained may he release his own emotions from control so that both together at the same moment may yield themselves for the final ecstatic flight.

Desire, which has been step by step intensified and heightened, is thus brought to a mutual fulfillment.

In this experience, as in all other phases of the difficult art of love, we must emphasize quality rather than quantity.

Complete love cannot be expressed merely in the number of times this communion is indulged in, but rather by the skill with which its highest fruits and creative joys are attained. All husbands and wives should remember that sex-communion should be considered as a true union of souls, not merely a physical function for the momentary relief of the sexual organs. Unless the psychic and spiritual desires are fulfilled, the relationship has been woefully deficient and the participants degraded and dissatisfied.

With this truth understood, the need for sex communion becomes more selective and less demanding. Because it brings into play the deeper nature and feelings of the participants, it takes on the nature of a sacrament. It must not therefore be sullied by crude levity or coarse frivolity, both of which defeat their own purpose.

When the threefold factors of human nature are brought into action, the sexual embrace not only satisfies but elevates both participants. The physical demands are harnessed for the expression of love. The woman who abhors the sexual act is usually the woman who has seen and felt it only in its selfishly physical aspects. Otherwise she would not be repelled by an activity of such manifold and life-giving possibilities.

We must, in conclusion, speak of the most neglected phase of the sex drama—that of *relaxation*. At the flight, body, mind and soul are brought together into the closest unity. "No more are they twain, but one flesh," in the words of the Bible. In this state of unconsciousness or superconsciousness they remain, until they both experience a drowsiness, a drop back to normal life. There is perhaps an impulse to sleep. Let us here point again to the diagram (page 128) which shows us that the descent of the woman's emotion is much slower and more gradual than that of the man. This means that the woman returns more slowly to a normal emotional condition after she has attained the orgasm.

Even when her desire is fully satisfied, this fact remains true. For certain women it requires at least fifteen or twenty minutes before the ecstasy of the emotional flight and climax has died down, whereas the average man relaxes at once and is overcome by drowsiness. This for the man is normal. The wife should forgive him if his interest in her seems suddenly to have vanished.

Nevertheless, continued consideration is far more desirable, if the skillful husband desires to round out with complete success the drama of love. He will notice that the affectionate nature of his wife now asserts itself anew. Passion is relaxed. Her emotions return almost through the same states in a descending scale to the normal, when she, too, falls into a peaceful slumber.

Even the completely satisfied wife is often unconscious of the effect of this final step upon her nature. This is the stage when she needs tenderness doubled and trebled. Her faculties are awake and intensely sensitive. She must be assured that the happiness, the joy and ecstasy they have experienced together have been the means of deepening his love which has not died out with physical gratification.

The skilled husband who possesses the art to remember the unspoken need of his wife in this stage, will be repaid by increased respect and love for his gentle manhood, by the closer unity of his marriage, the deepening beauty of his wife.

His tenderness should not cease with the end of the act. For in adding to the happiness of the woman he loves he will find his own more bountiful. Men who seek relief through the body of some unfortunate prostitute, hurry away from such women disillusioned and disgusted with themselves. Such an attitude toward a beloved wife is unspeakable. A wife senses this lack of respect even though it be concealed. Young husbands, through carelessness or thoughtlessness, are apt to fall into this error. I cannot too strongly warn them against such lack of reverence and to make their embrace of good-night or farewell lingeringly tender and brimming with reassurances of undying love.

Frivolity or levity, with a hurried performance and parting, will bring in some fashion its own penalty and punishment, and young couples are advised against the expression of any such attitude.

If possible it is desirable that husband and wife fall asleep in each other's arms, releasing the embrace only after the first refreshing slumber.

DEAR MRS. SANGER:

Your book entitled "Woman and the New Race" arrived yesterday and I have read it thru twice. You are truly doing a wonderful work for womankind. I am a victim of prudish parents. I was told nothing whatever of the facts of life. I did not even know where babies came from until I was a junior in high school. I was never a type to attract other children and I got no information thru this source. My father died before I finished high school and my mother worked in a factory. I worked outside school hours. I was ambitious to go thru college, so when my mother married a second time and went to California, I went to a neighboring town and worked for my board and room while going to college on a loan scholarship. I married a year before I finished college, not even knowing that I would be required to have physical unions with my husband. He was as patient as could be at first. Finally an aunt who has had six babies in nine years, told me what it would mean if I allowed my husband to have unions with me. So I have refused. We have lived together almost two years. I am growing more nervous and irritable all the time and have lost my appetite and fallen in weight. I am teaching. I must pay back the enormous debt I owe for my education, before I think of raising a family. My husband wants to start in business for himself. He can't so long as my school debt has to be paid. We have no home. I refuse to be made an incubator, as my poor aunt has been. Her health is almost ruined and her children do not receive proper care. My husband is growing more and more dissatisfied. He says he will leave if I do not allow him to have unions. I love him dearly and would be heartbroken if he should, but I will not subject myself to forced motherhood. I will not have children until I am ready for them, even if it means loosing the man I love. Mrs. Sanger, is there any way out? Can you give me the information which your book has made me see more clearly than ever, that I have a right to ask for? And can you help me to help my poor aunt who is expecting another child? I will do everything in my power to help you forward this cause. I am a college woman and a school teacher and if I can help you in any way please call upon me to do so.

Sincerely

Mrs. H. R. T.

CHAPTER X

THE RHYTHM OF SEX

"The permanence or periodicity of the sexual life must certainly affect the relations between the sexes."

"The type of periodicity, based on natural law or man-made habit—the former more conducive to permanence."

—Westermarck.

MANY people have been taught to look upon sexual intercourse merely as a physiological function. They consider love an appetite to be controlled yet to be regularly satisfied.

Attempts to regulate and systematize the time and place of sex-union in marriage have usually not been productive of happiness because what should be a source of ecstasy becomes a mere matter of habit, with duty instead of desire dictating the time and place.

Nevertheless the problem of mutual adjustment of desire must be met and solved. The successful solution of this problem depends as all others upon the proper and careful initiation, with adequate attention paid to every step toward the conquest of marital happiness.

In the first place, it is impossible to set hard and fast rules to be observed by every married couple. The age, the mental and physical constitution, the degree of stimulation, and many other factors must be considered. Sages and lawmakers from the dawn of humanity have insisted on the necessity of proper intervals between the acts of sexual communion. Mahomet prescribed eight days, Zoroaster nine days, both Solon and Socrates ten days, Moses forbade intercourse during the menstrual period and for a week following the cessation of the flow. In more modern times, Martin Luther, whose influence on the institution of modern marriage has been enormous, prescribed intercourse twice a week.

Customs of today are more or less a blend of the wisdom of past ages. It is generally conceded that over-indulgence and too rapid repetition of the act is harmful to both husband and wife.

Many men mistakenly believe that their virility is determined by the frequency in which they are able to indulge. Some of them even boast surreptitiously of this power.

Such a power misused and abused weakens the ability of sexual communion. There are three uses or purposes for sexual intercourse—physical relief, procreation and communion. The first two have little to do with the art of love. Power, says Balzac in his "Physiology of Love," does not consist in striking hard and often, but of striking properly.

Authorities are agreed that conservation of sexual powers *before* maturity and in the twenties preserves this energy and enables men to continue virile for a much longer period of years than when it is dissipated by excess through inability to control the appetite.

If the husband concerns himself with the quality of his performance instead of congratulating himself upon his vigor, which may, and in the majority of cases, does, leave the wife quite unsatisfied, he will soon find his own power and the consequent habit, paying greater dividends in health and joy, and in the increasing love for and of his mate.

Sexual experience can no longer be gauged by the number of "affairs" a man has had, either within or outside the bonds of matrimony. The man who is notoriously promiscuous is most often he who is unable to awaken the deeper love of any one woman. If the women's side of the story might be heard, we should undoubtedly hear a tale of selfishness, of disappointment, of this Don Juan's inability to understand anything but his own gluttonous appetite.

On the other hand, the intelligent monogamous husband with a wife whose love constantly deepens with the passing of the years, whose peaceful and poised countenance speaks louder than words the inner secret of sexual harmony and happiness—this is the man who is the master of love, and the real leader of humanity toward the future.

This problem of happiness in marriage cannot be satisfactorily solved except in blending the menstrual rhythm or periodicity in women with the other urges. Like the tides, there is an ebb and flow of sexual desire in normal women, and in some men. According to the cyclical theory of menstruation, the sexual desire in women consists of a series of wave-like periods determined by the monthly cycle. The menstrual cycle is complete in the normal woman every twenty-eight days, the period of menstruation taking up at least five of these.

Authorities and investigators are not in complete agreement upon the point when desire rises to its highest point. This undoubtedly varies in different women, according to age, climate and general environment. If fatigued, distressed or maladjusted and unhappy in her marriage relations, the full natural wave-like rhythm of desire is inhibited and often distorted.

Just what the period of desire might be could be found if our lives were not so stimulated and nerve-straining. The desire curve has no doubt been flattened out by excesses or sexual demands made upon the woman by ignorant but well-meaning husbands. Seldom does the married woman have the full control of her sex life, or having this, she is influenced by false suppositions concerning her husband's sexual needs, as well as by the custom of the ages of "wives submit yourselves unto your husbands."

Intelligent husbands should make a thoughtful study of the inner nature of their wives and seek to carry to consummation their own amorous desires on the rising movement of this wave instead of with its fall. If they do this, they may find themselves buoyed onward with the great sweep of a natural and possible cosmic rhythm, instead of fighting against a falling movement, when they find themselves in the position of a swimmer struggling against the tide. Such an intelligent study of the monthly cycle, which both intelligent mates should study and if possible keep a record of, would be an invaluable aid in the conquest of marital harmony, and the banishment of sexual discord which lies at the root of most unhappy marriages.

If the period of desire in women rises to a monthly acme, husband and wife might make of this period a renewed honeymoon of physical and spiritual communion. This, I believe everyone must agree, is infinitely preferable to making the act a routine function, indulged in as a duty and a habit.

To follow the counsel advised is conducive to making it a renewal, a discovery, a conquest of power. It also makes possible a long period of sexual relaxation, a season of sleeping and renewing powers. Monotonous regularity is fatal to a romantic spiritual union.

To study the more profound rhythm of life, to woo and win the woman anew each time is to preserve, to perpetuate the relationship and the romance.

It is also, from the point of view of the wife, the surest way to hold the interest of the husband and to intensify it.

Some have claimed that this hypothesis of the wave of rhythm in woman's sexual life has brought forth many premature conclusions and theories. In answer to this criticism, the immediate and obvious reply is that from every point of view thoughtfulness of the wife's cycles as well as of the longings of the husband makes married life more interesting, more stimulating, more poetic and infinitely more mysterious. It appeals to the intelligence as well as to the emotions.

To the objection that this theory and practice is merely substituting one habit of regularity for another, the answer would be that too little is yet known about the ebb and flow of woman's emotional life ever to suppose that the wave crest would be attained on a regular day each month. It would change perhaps from month to month, while the rhythm might be always at the foundation of this eternal and natural movement.

Marital relations based on this mating-season will, I am quite certain, do much toward the solution of many of the thorniest problems today, notably that of the so-called "frigidity" among women.

Undoubtedly many women today have lost consciousness of this monthly ebb and flow. It atrophies with woman's removal from the natural mode of life that prevails among savages and primitive tribes. Conditions of modern life, particularly of social life in cities, with increased nervous excitement, false stimulation and a hectic enslavement of hurry and speed is most likely to supersede and replace the tug and pull, the ebb and flow, of the great profound rhythms of life and nature.

Often a discord that results in neurasthenia, nervous collapse and general organic disorder is the result of the conflict between the primitive cycle or rhythm and the regularity accepted by custom.

To the objection that the habit of a monthly courtship and honeymoon between husband and wife would be to impose sexual restraint for too long a period on the man, the answer is this: most normal men, freed of that convention or self-deception which makes them hypocritically assume the position that they are

always at the acme of sexual power, so would
welcome this period of relaxation and pas-
sivity, and would resume the courtship with
more fiery ardor if their aggressive advances
were received or rejected on primitive or
biological impulses rather than on legal or
biblical codes.

The menstrual ebb and flow exists in the
woman of all races. It is curiously coincident
with the moon-cycle. Relatively men live on a
plane. In contrast, the physiological and emotional life of women tends to follow a wave-
like rhythm. Always a woman is on the
gradual upward or downward curve.

The highest peak of desire, which varies in
intensity and time in the individual is of the
very utmost importance in the sex life of the
woman. Every husband must bear it in mind
and take advantage of his study of the woman
whose happiness it should be his chief aim to
realize. No hard and fast rule can be set down
for the monthly rhythm, as like the breaking
waves on the shore, there is undoubtedly an
infinite variety and change. With some
women the wave motion may be more choppy,
a thing of great rise and fall, while with others,
it may be a slower, less accentuated motion.

The rise and fall of sexual desire is determined in the majority of cases by this wavelike rhythm. Havelock Ellis tells us in "Man and Woman" that in most healthy women the sexual emotions are strongest or at the maximum *before* the menstrual period, and at the lesser maximum after the period. It is more difficult to prove that mental vigor is also greatest at the same periods, but Ellis thinks this is extremely probable.

After the crest of the wave of vital activity is reached, or a day or two afterwards, the menstrual flow begins. This period is easily observable. It is the day or two preceding the menstrual period that women are mostly given, if they are at all predisposed to sudden caprices, fits of anger, nervousness, depressed and sad moods, impulses of jealousy. On the emotional side of their natures, there is more or less diminished self-control, they are more easily impressed. Menstruation and its difficulties permeate the whole being of a woman. It is especially necessary, therefore, that the husband understand this deep natural mystery and not aggravate her indisposition.

"This periodic discharge from the uterus, known as the menstrual flow, is a perfectly natural function of the body, and should not be regarded as an 'illness.'"

The husband should learn to respond to this cycle, to take advantage of her exact condition in this moon-monthly rhythm instead of beginning his lovemaking at the wrong period. He must, in short, fall into step with her movement instead of combating and disturbing it. This latter behavior can only produce conflict and discord.

Among all intelligent couples, it is possible and it is highly advisable that the wife indicate her own desire in this matter if she has learned to become conscious of the wave-like ebb and flow of her own emotions.

According to the diagram in Ellis' "Man and Woman," there would be two intervals for communion during the moon month of twenty-eight days; at the wave crest before the menstrual flow, and after it, an interval of about eleven days. Following this there would be a respite or sexual relaxation of about two weeks or sixteen days.

At these periods, mutual desire would set the number of times for cohabitation. There would need to be no restraint exercised except that imposed by lack of desire.

Thus, in women in whom the monthly cycle is more pronounced this periodicity would be more or less evident. In those in whom it is scarcely noticeable, this hypothesis might develop and strengthen this tendency.

Sex love instead of becoming a habit for physical relief, would be allowed to take on more of the thrill and excitement of dramatic activity. No longer would it be a matter of mere routine, but should partake of the great tidal rhythm of nature. No longer would it be determined by the appetite of one participant alone, but would be enhanced and made doubly adventurous by the ceaseless search for higher and more thrilling ecstasy.

DEAR MRS. SANGER:

My sorrows are not too many children, but they are just as great. I want children, always have wanted children and have been denied them. I am not strong, have always had poor health since girlhood. I am 30 years old and have been married eight years. I can write my troubles to you, for I feel you will understand and help me and tell me if I am right or wrong. My husband does not want children. He does not satisfy me and I cannot respond. Never in my eight years of married life have I responded. I am so unhappy about it and I know I am not normal, or I would not be this way. Is it that I could not have children or is it because of disorders of my womb or ovaries. I never had courage to go to a doctor and I never have talked with other women on sex problems.

My menstrual periods are always long and often times too soon. Your Chapter on Continence, I didn't fully understand. It is written in plain every day language —but does continence mean such intercourse as I have or does it mean no intercourse at all?

If you are allowed to give such information through letters will be thankful for it. If medicine will make me well and normal, I want to know what to use. If we were sure I would not get pregnant, would I be natural, could I respond?

MRS. E. B.

CHAPTER XI

PSYCHIC IMPOTENCE AND FRIGIDITY

AGAIN and again I have emphasized the
need of adequate preparation, complete
avoidance of hurry and nervousness. This is
a real need, physiological as well as emotional.
The accessories of the act, the wooing, the romance, the tuning in,—all fulfill a definite
physiological function.

Swept off their feet by uncontrolled ecstasy,
mastered by their passions, aiming only for the
immediate gratification of desire, many men
find themselves suddenly and inexplicably be-
reft of the power to continue. This phenome-
non may be the result of an acute and even an
unconscious nervousness, of too great a nervous tension. The young man may even be
virile, healthy and vigorous, an ardent lover;
and yet, at the great moment, while emotional
desire runs high, the erection has relaxed.

This is a most embarrassing situation for the
young husband and for his bride as well. This

defeat, and the chagrin created by it, may lead to a more or less permanent period of impotence. If experienced, the man may have some knowledge of this temporary impotence. If he is lacking in experience, he may imagine that he had lost his manhood, that he cannot fulfill his duty, and that the woman he has loved will believe him impotent. All of these thoughts increase and intensify his anxiety. He may lose all confidence in himself. His imagination and his belief may make this impotence of longer duration. In desperation he may make vain attempts to fulfil his part. But each attempt increases his exhaustion and adds to his defeat.

In such a situation, all such attempts are useless. At this point the bride should recognize that there is no occasion for alarm, that the proper emotional rhythm has not yet been established, that the culmination of the nuptial act must be postponed to another time. Therefore she should not only urge her husband to rest but also assure him anew of her love and confidence. Often when the wife has assumed this attitude (instead of expressing her own disappointment) by assuming the active part in reassuring the husband, through her caresses and tender understanding, she reawakens the nervous and emotional fires. Relaxation and rest are the only remedies for temporary psychic impotence on the part of the husband.

Often such a condition is a danger signal that the act has been indulged in too often, especially in the earlier periods of marriage.

In some cases, however, the long continued habit of masturbation renders young men partially impotent. If this practice is prolonged the man may discover that while erection may occur as the result of his own imaginations and sensations, the thought or the touch of his wife has lost its power to cause a sufficiently strong erection to carry out the act of intercourse. In some cases he may not be sexually stimulated at all. In other cases, erection may occur but relapse almost immediately.

One case of a young man who had indulged in the practice of masturbation merely for physical relief was brought to my attention. He married and no more than one week after the ceremony his bride came weeping to me, asking for advice. She confided that the young husband's attempts at intercourse were revolting to her, as well as disturbing to her nervous system. Because she wished to have a family, she was crushed by grief at the predicament in which she found herself, for she was in love with the man of her choice. Above everything else I recommended her to be patient, sympathetic and to do everything in her power to reassure him of her confidence. Both were nervous, frightened, and thrown into the deepest chagrin. Rest and emotional relaxation were needed, and no attempts at intercourse should even be attempted for several weeks. Intimacy and affection and knowledge of each other was in this case the first essential. I advised the young woman that all the outgoing streams of affection and confidence should be strengthened before the final act of sex communion should be thought of again.

The husband should, of course, make a determined effort to free himself of the pernicious habit which had caused this temporary tragedy, and which had such a deleterious effect upon his nerve centers.

The advice was followed and within six months not only had this marriage been successfully consummated, but a baby was on its way into the world. By a strict adherence to the simple rules advised, by the wife's tactful sympathy—complete potency was regained and with it an added ambition and marital understanding.

Another case of impotence through masturbation was brought to my attention. But in this case the young man indulged not merely for physical relief. His imagination was fired by feminine attire, by magazine covers. His imagination had been perverted and fixed by the practice, and he failed to break through the slavery of the habit.

So-called psychic impotence in men is brought about through the protracted habit of masturbation, by excessive indulgence in sexual intercourse, and very often by disturbing environments, nervous tension, fear or anxiety, or alcohol. There is likewise a corresponding condition in women, rendering impossible or unsatisfactory the act of sex communion. Among many women this state of "frigidity" is brought about either by a complete indifference and lack of desire, or when passion is present by the inability of her partner to coax this passion to its highest and culminating point.

The reasons for this condition are as various

as the different types of "frigid" women. Among certain women the desire for sexual contact is strong, but they confess themselves constitutionally unable to reach an orgasm. Other women confess that they have no desire for sexual union at all, and that the act is even repulsive to them. They are affectionate, responsive to the caresses of their husbands, but derive no joy from sex contact. These are the two main types of "frigid" women found in the Anglo-Saxon countries today. There are, of course, many individual cases that fall outside these two main groups. But few women are absolutely and pathologically frigid.

I have sought to show in a previous chapter that women are as a rule constitutionally unable to reach the climax of the drama of love at the same time as men. But this does not mean that women on this account are to be classified as "frigid."

Many women have never experienced the supreme moment of the love drama because of the husband's extreme disregard for her and his ignorance of her emotional nature during coitus. He fails to control his own passions and is interested only in the immediate gratification of his own desire. His lack of consideration for the needs of his wife, who experiences no joy in the act, since she is merely the passive receptacle of her husband's passion, leads her to believe that she is "cold."

We cannot too strongly emphasize the necessity of young husbands studying the emotional needs of their wives, for it is upon this art that the foundations of married love are based. It is out of this ability, developed and strengthened (and an endless source of vitality gained) that enduring happiness in marriage grows.

The second and larger group of so-called "cold" women are those in whom desire still remains sleeping. In these women sex desire is not present because it has never been awakend. Affection is present, and human affection is important, but until the woman experiences positive sex desire she remains in a "frigid" state.

The husband must therefore do everything in his power to fan the flame of desire in his loved one. He must seek to get rid of the inhibitions, the fears or anxiety which hold her back from complete enjoyment.

Certain women, for instance, are so sensitive to noises that the slightest sound, in the next room or in any part of the house, which penetrates the atmosphere, destroys her enjoyment. Thus this thought, the product of fear and anxiety, restrains and suppresses desire, so that whatever the husband does, he cannot bring it to a climax. Too frequent demands are another cause that destroys the desire among some women. The nervous system in women is a delicate and intricate mechanism and is subject to fatigue. Overstimulation, excesses, indulgence in intercourse in season and out, all bring sexual fatigue and even positive repulsion, especially to a highly sensitive woman who has not yet been fully awakened. To indulge in too frequent intercourse under such conditions becomes distasteful to her. It becomes more and more difficult to bring on an orgasm and, eventually, in certain cases, quite impossible.

Factors influencing sex desire are food, health, sleep, music, happiness, alcohol, as well as frequently of act, completeness of organism, worry, anxiety, sorrow and fear of pregnancy.

In all cases of so-called frigidity, special attention should be paid to the facts recounted in Chapters VIII and IX and complete time, attention and precautions taken. Among these are:

Establish conditions of complete isolation, privacy, and leisure. Remove all things which would cause fear and worry.

Let the husband encourage his wife to relax herself completely, so that her love may find complete expression.

Win and woo each time anew.

CHAPTER XII
SETTLING DOWN

Texas.

DEAR MRS. SANGER:

I wonder if you could help me solve my problems, too. It is not "wrong teaching" that causes my aversions to sexual relations with my husband, for I had no teaching whatever. Never-the-less, my indifference to same is about to disrupt our home—I love my husband, and desire very much to enjoy martial relations with him; but find no real pleasure in it, and never have, though I have endured it for eight years and have borne two fine children. For their sakes, can't you help me preserve our home?

MRS. W. H. M.

CHAPTER XII

SETTLING DOWN

"What is it men in women do require?
The lineaments of satisfied desire.
What is it women do in men require?
The lineaments of gratified desire."
—*William Blake.*

THE honeymoon is the period during which the young wife and husband establish mutual adjustment and spiritual harmony.

The period which follows is more difficult.

The problem during the first two or three years of married life is how to keep romance alive in spite of the influence of the prosaic demands of everyday life. How to make love and romance the crowning power to success instead of a hindrance.

The first few years of married life are difficult because of the multitude of pressing problems they thrust upon young wives and husbands.

First of all, these years are usually ones of great economic stress, particularly for husbands whose salaries are small. The young man is making a great effort to establish himself in his work, his business, his profession. He often needs all the capital he has to get himself established. If he is ambitious, he is putting tremendous energy in his work, hoping thus to provide comforts and luxuries for his wife and the family-to-be.

If this is the case, the husband is liable to fall into the "tired business man" psychology, to return to his home in the evening worn-out by his work or his struggles during the day for an economic footing. Love should increase his efficiency, self-assurance and ambition. Or, if his economic problem is already solved and there are no serious financial worries, the young couple may seek hectic diversions in what is known as "the younger married set," as though afraid to remain in each other's company. This endless gregariousness of social gaiety, dinners and country clubs, is often a symptom of no community of deep interests, and often it gives rise to temptations, quarrels and jealousies which unite to destroy the romance of a couple for whom during the honeymoon life was full of promise.

Or happiness in marriage during these years
may be wrecked by fear—in many young wives
the fear of pregnancy. This fear becomes a
reality. She becomes a mother before she is
ready to have a family. Young, full of life,
entitled to develop to maturity this love and
romance, many young wives who enter matrimony with bright dreams of the future, find
themselves all too soon slaves to children,
slaves to poverty, slaves to the never-ending
rounds of household toil. Romance cannot
live or bloom where fear and discontent thrive
like weeds.

This is the great central problem of the
young married couple and is discussed in a
later chapter.

The important aim during the earlier years
of marriage must be to live out this romance,
to discover in marital love a source of renewed
energy and vitality, a reservoir of self-
confidence, mutual aid and spiritual and physical vigor.

In order to bring this about, mutual love
must be protected, cultivated, rejuvenated and
constantly refreshed. While it must be made
a part of the whole of life, it should be looked
upon as the source, the ever-freshening foun-

tain from which strength is derived. It is for this reason that, like all growing organisms, love must be tenderly cherished and cultivated if it is going to bear the fruit of continued happiness.

Certain times, certain periods, must therefore be held sacred to love. Every outward gesture, every ceremonious act, every formality through which this deep, inner love finds external expression, must be carefully observed, not merely as an empty duty, but as a symbol.

I am not one of those who believe that once embarked on the sea of matrimony, all personal boundaries should be cast aside, or that personal privacy should be discarded.

Easy familiarity, invasion of personal and individual rights, or impositions on the good nature of those with whom one lives in the most intimate associations—such actions as these growing into habits, are bound to cause the greatest unhappiness. It is therefore advisable to arrange the living arrangements, in so far as it is possible and practical—so neither husband nor wife may slip unconsciously into a relationship that wears down the velvety surface of romance and love to that of threadbare habit.

Petty quarrels, bickerings and disagreements over details non-essential may become a habit. When they do, a separation, at least a spiritual separation, has already taken place. And a separation of the heart is more injurious to love than a physical separation. Petty quarrels inevitably lead to more serious ones. They may be patched up, patched up again and again, yet each quarrel is a mar on the perfect weaving of two lives, which marriage should be in reality as well as in theory.

More tact is needed in adjusting the relationship between husband and wife than in less intimate relations. Tact is quite compatible with frankness and honesty. A certain amount of individual privacy should be made possible in every home, for both husband and wife. In these days of high rents and crowded apartments, this is not seemingly possible. Yet if this need is foreseen and discussed frankly at the beginning, if this right is openly recognized, misunderstanding may later be avoided.

Let the wife keep alive the innate modesty natural to a normal woman. Do not allow the performance of daily acts of hygiene in the husband's presence, dressing and undressing, hair curling, teeth cleaning, etc., for careless exposure of body lessens the effect its beauty has on the husband. Try to avoid that slump in the relationship, where each "gets used" to all those little tendernesses and charms which at first were a source of stimulation and delight. Keep intact all the gifts of love for the great drama. Don't scatter heedlessly the charms that should be reserved for a special time and place. See that your love life is the source of your health life.

Those who have failed in marital life to discover the inexhaustible source of energy and life-giving power to be derived from happiness in marriage have at their command only a small part of the power which they actually possess and which is released through sexual expression.

Energies which slumber deep within one's nature are called forth into human activity by this power of love. This is true in a real sense, and in no mere poetic or sentimental fashion.

Unhappy people are notoriously listless and inefficient or nervous in the workaday world. And the maximum of happiness and poise is attainable only from the reservoir of love, the communion of sex.

The man who has found enduring and cumulating happiness in his marriage relation, who has freed himself of the hampering inhibitions that destroy his confidence in himself, and has found increased strength and courage in this living relationship, is spurred on to make full use of his mental and physical resources.

Living life to the full, exercising the full emotional life, one is less liable to disease, neurasthenia or depression.

But sex-love and happiness in marriage, I repeat, do not just happen. This love is a plant that must be carefully nurtured and cultivated.

Eternal vigilance is the price of marital happiness. Therefore the young husband must never let his relation with his wife sink to the level of routine habit, of everyday monotony. He will refreshen the romance by gifts and surprises. No matter how limited his income, no matter how tiring his work, he will never place a higher value on the external things of life than upon this, the eternal source of his power and strength.

Men in many cases destroy the marriage relation by allowing it to drift into a sort of master-slave relation—the relation out of which modern marriage has at last managed to elevate itself. But the master-slave relation is sometimes as much the wife's fault as the husband's.

Therefore in the initial conference when such things are decided, unpleasant or disagreeable tasks and household duties should not be turned over to the wife. Such tasks shared equally become unimportant. Bearing them alone they become burdens.

The nuptial relation must be kept romantic. When either feels that fatigue or monotony is beginning to enter the relation, he or she must take the initiative of intensifying and rejuvenating it, instead of merely complaining of the behavior of the other. There are a hundred possible ways of breaking the habitual routine, of surprising the mate into a fresh realization that he or she is taking too much for granted.

Every human being—it is one of the weaknesses of human nature—naturally tends to form habits. This is perhaps truer of the marriage relation than of any other. And it is habit that kills romance rather than faithlessness or fickleness.

Love, like every other function, must be exercised, translated into action, in order that it may grow and develop. Most people are too likely nowadays to suppress the outward expression of this emotion. Constantly inhibited or suppressed the emotion dies a long lingering death. Therefore, since love is the most valuable emotion given to human beings, they must seek to express it. Unclamp this emotion; let it have full, healthy exercise. Let it express itself in words, in gestures, in actions. Dramatize your love whenever possible, however possible. It will repay you many times and it will grow strong according to the exercise it is given.

Do not be afraid to take the brakes off your heart, to surrender yourself to love. Neither spiritually nor physically can love thrive when it is subject always to fear, tension and strain. That is why there should be more of the spirit of play in the marital relation.

It would be a good rule to make at the beginning of marriage, and to follow with the same regularity that is given over to personal hygiene or any of the wholesome, normal functions of life, that a certain number of hours daily should be given over to this intimate seclusion of husband and wife during which they may play together, to delight in each other's presence, to leave aside the duties and thoughts of business and expenses, to probe beneath the outward surface of each other's nature and thus to arrive at a full understanding of each other and the nature of the spiritual bond which unites one with the other.

"Lovers in their play," says Havelock Ellis, "are moving amongst the highest human activities, alike of the body and of the soul. They are passing to each other the sacramental chalice of that wine which imparts the deepest joy men and women can know. They are subtly weaving the invisible cords that bind husband and wife together more truly and more firmly than the priest of any church."

DEAR MRS. SANGER,—

In the first place I only wish I had been able to get in touch with your work years ago. It might have saved my home, as it is I am a very unhappy woman working more than my strength is equal to, to raise my children alone, being separated from my husband, after bearing 9 children to him, unwilling mostly, 8 of which are living. He being a very strong, sexually, I mean as well as otherwise, I being delicate found bearing children far too much for me, and being married young at 18 years, ignorant of any means of preventing pregnancy. Had my children very fast. Consequently we drifted apart. Circumstances going from bad to worse, he taking to gambling, refusing to work, only hate and misery, trouble and unpleasantness, I trying to support the family by maternity nursing often with one little one with me, and at the same time pregnant. As time wore on he became more disagreeable and put some of the children from home and the others would leave as they grew up. So I was obliged to leave him, taking the six little children with me, the two eldest were taking care of themselves. I have struggled on for 4 years now. I still have 4 children under 14, one not 6 yet. I find it very hard to make ends meet sometimes. I have one daughter married, and one about to be married. My son, only one, is 22, and so very much like all the faults in his father. I fear for his future. I struggled hard to give him a good education, and he don't make any use of it, going from one thing to another, barely supporting himself and refusing to help me in any way to raise the family. One girl of 18 is anemic, and under treatment just now. Now I am going to ask you to put me in touch with some means of Birth

Control for my daughters. I would go a long ways to save them a life like mine. I would rather follow any of them to their graves than to live a life of suffering like I have lived, nothing but disappointment in the tender loving ways I had such great hopes of. Thanking you in advance and wishing your work God's Speed, and blessing, for I do see so much happiness can come to so many people. My heart just aches for them lest they should share my kind of troubles. May God forbid such. Please reply.

Sincerely,

Mrs. S. A. S.

CHAPTER XIII

PREMATURE PARENTHOOD AND WHY TO AVOID IT

COMING together with widely differing likes and dislikes, varying inheritances and often with widely divergent training and ideals, the two young people who marry will not be long in discovering that they may have much less in common than they had ever dreamed possible.

When Society has tossed them a marriage certificate and the Church has concluded the ceremony which has legally united them, they are then forced back upon their own resources. Society, so to speak, has washed its hands of the young couple, or cast this man and this woman into the deep waters of matrimony, where they are left to sink or swim as best they may.

The certificate of marriage solves nothing. Rather it accentuates the greater and more complex problems of life. To find a solution to this great problem of living together and growing together requires all the combined intelligence and foresight both man and woman can command. Drifting into this relation will offer no solution, for very often those who drift into marriage, drift out of it in the same aimless fashion.

Others, who have not realized that the marriage of a man and woman is not merely a legal sanction for parenthood, but that it is an important relation in itself—the most important one in human life—often find themselves defeated and forced into an accidental and premature parenthood for which they are not financially or spiritually prepared.

Two years at least are necessary to cement the bonds of love and to establish the marriage relation. Parenthood should therefore be postponed by every young married couple until at least the third year of marriage.

Why is this advisable?

When the young wife is forced into maternity too soon, both are cheated out of marital adjustment and harmony that require time to mature and develop. The plunge into parenthood prematurely with all its problems and disturbances, is like the blighting of a bud before it has been given time to blossom.

Even in the fully matured healthy wife pregnancy has a disturbing physiological and nervous reaction. Temporarily the whole character and temperament of the woman undergoes profound changes. Usually nausea, headaches, irritability, loss of appetite, ensue. At the beginning of this period there develop temporary eccentricities that do not belong to the woman in her normal condition.

If the bride is enforced into an unwilling or accidental pregnancy during the honeymoon or the early stages of their marital love, the young husband is deprived of the possible opportunity of knowing his wife during one of the most interesting stages of her development. He has known her in the exciting days of courtship and during the heightened though brief period of the honeymoon, and now, alas, she enters all too soon the ominous days of early pregnancy. Never under such conditions can he know her in the growing beauty and ripening of mature womanhood. He has known her as a romantic girl before marriage —and now as a mother-to-be, frightened, timorous, and physically and nervously upset by the great ordeal she must go through.

Here often begins a spiritual separation between husband and wife. Conscious of his own helplessness, likewise of his own responsibility, the young husband feels it his duty to leave her alone. This enforced separation is spiritual rather than physical. Outwardly the relation may seem the same. It may be a separation only in the sense that no real unity or welding has been attained. Engrossed by this new problem, the young wife may resign herself to the inevitable and enters a state of passive resignation that is deadening to her love-life. She is in no condition to enjoy companionship. Beneath the superficial and conventional expression of happiness at the approaching parenthood, there may rankle a suppressed resentment at the young husband's careless pride in becoming a father. The young bride knows that she is paying too great a price for the brief and happy days of her honeymoon. She has been swept too rapidly from girlhood to motherhood. Love and romance, as many young wives have confessed to me, were but traps leading her to endless travail and enslavement. And this hidden rankling is often directed toward the husband, whom the wife holds responsible for her accidental pregnancy.

This unhappy condition would not have occurred if they had time to become one, if there were a period of two years during which the bonds of love might be firmly cemented, for time alone can produce this unity. It is a process of growth. Married love does not spring fullgrown into life. It is a delicate plant and it grows from the seed. It must be deeply and firmly rooted, nourished by the sunlight of tenderness, courtship and mutual consideration, before it can produce fine flowers and fruits. This period is as essential for human development as the period of body-building and adolescence.

It is a period of mutual adjustment. It is a period of spiritual discovery and exploration, of finding one's self and one's beloved. It is a period for the full and untroubled expression of passionate love. It is a period for cultural development. It thrusts forward its own complex problems—problems, let it be understood, intricately complex in themselves.

Husband and wife must solve many problems only by *living through them,* not by any cut and dried rules and regulations. For marriage brings with it problems that are individual and unique for each couple.

If instead of solving these problems of early

parenthood, in which the life of a third person is immediately involved, a child thrusts itself into the lives of young husband and wife, these fundamental problems of marriage are never given the attention they deserve. A new situation arises, and in innumerable cases, love, as the old adage has it, flies out of the window.

We must recognize that the whole position of womanhood has changed today. Not so many years ago it was assumed to be a just and natural state of affairs that marriage was considered as nothing but a preliminary to motherhood. A girl passed from the guardianship of her father or nearest male relative to that of her husband. She had no will, no wishes of her own. Hers not to question why, but merely to fulfil duties imposed upon her by the man into whose care she was given.

Marriage was synonymous with maternity. But the pain, the suffering, the wrecked lives of women and children that such a system caused, show us that it did not work successfully. Like all other professions, motherhood must serve its period of apprenticeship.

Today women are on the whole much more individual. They possess as strong likes and dislikes as men. They live more and more on

the plane of social equality with men. They
are better companions. We should be glad
that there is more enjoyable companionship
and real friendship between men and women.

This very fact, it is true, complicates the
marriage relation, and at the same time en-
nobles it. Marriage no longer means the
slavish subservience of the woman to the will
of the man. It means, instead, the union of
two strong and highly individualized natures.
Their first problem is to find out just what the
terms of this partnership are to be. Understanding full and complete cannot come all at
once, in one revealing flash. It takes time
to arrive at a full and sympathetic understanding of each other, and mutually to arrange
lives to increase this understanding. Out of
the mutual adjustments, harmony must grow
and discords gradually disappear.

These results cannot be obtained if the problem of parenthood is thrust upon the young
husband and wife before they are spiritually
and economically prepared to meet it. For
naturally the coming of the first baby means
that all other problems must be thrust aside.
That baby is a great fact, a reality that must
be met. Preparations must be made for its

coming. The layette must be prepared. The doctor must be consulted. The health of the wife may need consideration. The young mother will probably prefer to go to the hospital. All of these preparations are small compared to the régime after the coming of the infant.

Now there is a proper moment for every human activity, a proper season for every step in self-development. The period for cementing the bond of love is no exception to this great truth. For only by the full and glorious living through these years of early marriage are the foundations of an enduring and happy married life rendered possible. By this period the woman attains a spiritual freedom. Her womanhood has a chance to bloom. She wins a mastery over her destiny; she acquires self-reliance, poise, strength, a youthful maturity. She abolishes fear. Incidentally, few of us realize, since the world keeps no record of this fact, how many human beings are conceived in fear and even in repugnance by young mothers who are the victims of undesired maternity. Nor has science yet determined the possibilities of a generation conceived and born of *conscious* desire.

In the wife who has lived through a happy marriage, for whom the bonds of passionate love have been fully cemented, maternal desire is intensified and matured. Motherhood becomes for such a woman not a penalty or a punishment, but the road by which she travels onward toward completely rounded self-development. Motherhood thus helps her toward the unfolding and realization of her higher nature.

Her children are not mere accidents, the outcome of chance. When motherhood is a mere accident, as so often it is in the early years of careless or reckless marriages, a constant fear of pregnancy may poison the days and nights of the young mother. Her marriage is thus converted into a tragedy. Motherhood becomes for her a horror instead of a joyfully fulfilled function.

Millions of marriages have been blighted, not because of any lack of love between the young husband and wife, but because children have come too soon. Often these brides become mothers before they have reached even physical maturity, before they have completed the period of adolescence. This period in our race is as a rule complete around the age of twenty-three. Motherhood is possible after the first menstruation. But what is physically possible is very often from every other point of view inadvisable. A young woman should be fully matured from every point of view—physically, mentally and psychically before maternity is thrust upon her.

Those who advise early maternity neglect the spiritual foundation upon which marriage must inevitably be built. This takes time. They also ignore the financial responsibility a family brings.

The young couple begin to build a home. They may have just enough to get along together. The young wife, as in so many cases of early marriage these days, decides to continue her work. They are partners in every way—a commendable thing. The young man is just beginning his career—his salary is probably small. Nevertheless, they manage to get along, their hardships are amusing, and are looked upon as fun. Then suddenly one day, the young wife announces her pregnancy. The situation changes immediately. There are added expenses. The wife must give up her work. The husband must go into debt to pay the expenses of the new and joyfully received arrival. The novelty lasts for some time. The young wife assumes the household duties and the ever growing care of the infant. For a time the child seems to bring the couple closer together. But more often there ensues a concealed resentment on the part of the immature mother at the constant drudgery and slavery to the unfortunate child who has arrived too early upon the scene, which has interfered with her love life.

Two brothers I know married practically at the same time. They were both carpenters, living in the same neighborhood. The wife of the one gave birth to six children in a period of ten years. In spite of the efforts of the man to sustain the family, they were forced at the end of ten years to accept outside charity. The wife became a household drudge, nervous, broken, spiritless, neglected by her husband, despised by her children. The wife of the other brother did not become a mother until three years after marriage. This man remained throughout the ten years of my observation, clean, alert, honest, kind to his wife and two children. The wife kept up neat, tidy looks and was able to help her husband and children to advance themselves. Yet at the time of marriage both girls were equally attractive and intelligent.

The problem of premature parenthood is intensified and aggravated when a second infant follows too rapidly the advent of the first, and inevitably husband and wife are made the slaves of this undreamed of situation, bravely trying to stave off poverty, whipped to desperation by the heavy hand of chance and involuntary parenthood. How can they then recapture their early love? It is not surprising that more often they do not even trouble themselves to conceal the contempt which is the bitter fruit of that young and romantic passion.

For the unthinking husband, the "proud papa," the blushing bride is converted at once into the "mother of my children." It is not an unusual occurrence to find that three months after the birth of the baby, the parents are thinking and speaking to each other as "mumsy" and "daddy." The lover and sweetheart relation has disappeared forever and the "mama-papa" relation has taken its place.

Instead of being a self-determined and self-directing love, everything is henceforward determined by the sweet tyranny of the child.

I know of several young mothers, despite a great love for the child, to rebel against this intolerable situation. Vaguely feeling that this new maternity has rendered them unattractive to their husbands, slaves to deadly routine of bottles, baths and washing, they have revolted. I know of innumerable marriages which have been wrecked by premature parenthood.

Love has ever been blighted by the coming of children before the real foundations of marriage have been established. Quite aside from the injustice done to the child who has been brought accidentally into the world, this lamentable fact sinks into insignificance when compared to the injustice inflicted by chance upon the young couple, and the irreparable blow to their love occasioned by premature or involuntary parenthood.

For these reasons, in order that harmonious and happy marriage may be established as the foundation for happy homes and the advent of healthy and desired children, premature parenthood must be avoided. Birth Control is the instrument by which this universal problem may be solved.

DEAR MRS. SANGER:

My wife with our two little daughters live in ———,
while I have been separated from them a year, having
started for ——— last February. I cannot help but
feel that the separation would never have occurred had
I known 10 years ago what I know now about sex
matters. Of the hundreds of dollars paid to doctors
for my wife's illness, it is now my conviction that fully
98% would have been unnecessary had we the proper
knowledge of our bodies and contraceptives; to say
nothing of the suffering and misunderstandings result-
ing from our lack of this knowledge. We are now
considering a reconciliation, as there has been no divorce,
no poverty, and no public knowledge of our "trial divorce." We have simply been living 2400 miles apart
for a year.

There is no disease in our family as both of us have
always been chaste. We are of equal age and education
and mental capacity. Sex ignorance seems to have been
the rock on which our matrimonial ship grounded. Perhaps you can help to float the good ship again. But
the best interests of our 2 girls of course demand that
we live together, I think we can do this in harmony if
we can secure reliable and complete contraceptive information. I know enough about my own body to live
in good health and physical condition under any ordinary circumstances. It is in behalf of my wife that
I am now writing to you. I am willing to assume any
risk to enable her to get this information, whether it
be from America, Holland or Australia, as I am certain
that all women are entitled to it.

D. H. K.

CHAPTER XIV

BIRTH CONTROL IN PRACTICE

WE have seen from our last chapter that from the point of view of all concerned —husband, wife and child—the control of the generative function, especially during the earlier years of marriage—recommends itself to intelligent and prudent couples who have their own well-being and that of their future families at heart. Birth control is a scientific practice which permits young husbands and wives to guide and direct their own destinies and to build up their health, happiness and economic strength.

Unfortunately the laws of the United States have not yet been amended to allow me to write as fully upon this subject as I should like to, nor do they permit me to state the method or methods I consider safest, wisest and most harmless.

Nevertheless I shall try to warn against uncertain and often dangerous methods advocated and practiced in this country today which do not fulfil requirements and which should, for various reasons, be discontinued. From my experience and knowledge of women who apply to me for help, I wish to emphasize the absolute necessity for each wife and mother desirous of obtaining safe and hygienic knowledge of birth control to apply to her regular physician. Information picked up from neighbors or intimate women friends, no matter how helpful their intentions may be, is not to be relied upon. What advice may be helpful for one may be useless for another.

Let us also acknowledge at the outset that the science of Birth Control has until the present day not been correlated with the practice of medicine. Consequently this science has not been standardized. While the majority of educated and intelligent classes in every civilized country of the world have practised birth control in one form or another during the present century and many of them for the past one hundred years, there are no scientific records or data concerning this practice, or of the success or failure of any particular method of birth control.

The practical phase of birth control has been advanced for the most part on theory or by word of mouth, by very limited personal experience rather than by the collection and testing of data from wider sources. Acknowledging this fact, we must realize the importance of proceeding slowly in the advocacy of any particular or general methods of contraception.

However, on the basis of our admittedly limited studies, certain facts nevertheless stand out clearly:

1. There is no one method of contraception that is suitable to be used by all men or women.

2. A method which may be of the utmost satisfaction in one case may be an utter and absolute failure in another.

3. One woman should not recommend to another any special method of prevention. Each woman is individual and needs special advice by a physician.

4. A physical examination is the best, preliminary step toward ascertaining the suitable method of birth control in each individual case.

5. The use and direction of the method should be determined by the wife rather than the husband. This is necessary to safeguard the health of both.

6. The two methods generally used by men

are known to be unsatisfactory to many men and to their wives likewise.

7. A douche, whether of cold water or an antiseptic solution, cannot be relied upon as a contraceptive. It is only a cleansing agent, and should in no sense be relied upon for the prevention of conception.

8. The superstition that during the period of nursing a baby the mother is safe from conceiving another is not true in fact.

9. The "safe period" recommended by the Roman Catholic Church and by certain physicians as a period in the month during which the wife does not conceive, is not to be relied upon.

10. The interuterine instruments are strongly condemned by the most experienced members of the medical profession and by the Clinical Research Department of the American Birth Control League.

11. The safest and most hygienic methods known today cannot be used by the unmarried girl.

These are the facts, directly and simply told. They may be of little use to the mother already distracted and worried from too frequent pregnancy and childbearing. She may throw aside this book, exclaiming: "I know all these things already! Why doesn't she tell me of something I can use, something that will help me out of my predicament?"

Such a woman should know that even were I to tell here what are known to be successful and reliable methods of contraception, it would be unsafe for women to act upon that advice without first consulting her physician, midwife or obstetrical nurse. For each woman must ascertain what is best suitable to her own physical needs and physiological structure.

It should never be forgotten that every woman differs in her physiological and bodily make-up. The bride-to-be cannot be given the same advice as the mother of a small family. The mother of nine or ten children presents a case entirely different from the woman who has given birth to but one or two.

Similarly, the mother who has always had sound medical attention and care before, during and after the birth of her babies presents an entirely different problem from that of the unfortunate woman whose womb is torn and lacerated.

Furthermore, the woman who can afford the luxury of remaining in the hospital for ten days, or even two or three weeks after the birth of her infant, is, it goes without saying, not to be given the same advice as the poor mother who has arisen the same day to perform household duties, or has had to return almost immediately to factory or shop to earn bread for the hungry mouths of her ever-increasing family.

In short, to secure reliable advice concerning her individual condition, each woman should undergo a physical examination by a physician in whom she has fullest confidence. If your family physician refuses this advice, do not on this account give up. Try again and again until you find a physician who understands your case and can advise you according to your individual needs.

Advice given in books or pamphlets, reliable as it may be for the majority of women, cannot be relied upon as a certainty that can be practiced by all. It may give results safe and sure, 100 per cent. perfect for one hundred women; and yet the methods advocated may fail—*you*. Why? Because your womb may be tipped forward or backward. Or it may hang too low in the vaginal canal. Or it may be very high in the vaginal canal and out of reach of the means of protection advised. There are many reasons why the method best suited to certain women may be unsuited and unfit for others.

Successfully to prevent conception means eternal vigilance. You cannot afford to overlook the necessary precaution even once. One mistake or laxness in a year may result in a possible pregnancy each year. Yet the precautions which may seem irksome at first soon become a matter of course and hygiene. Be constantly careful and prepare for each act of intercourse as accurately as a surgeon would prepare for an operation. The surgeon knows that the slightest carelessness may render his work valueless and may cost the life or future health of the patient he is operating upon.

To prevent pregnancy hygienic and careful preliminary precautions must also be taken.

Some women who find themselves pregnant are too ready to blame the method advised, when, as a matter of fact, they have been careless in applying it or temporarily negligent. In almost every case in which the woman is truthful, she admits that perhaps "just once" as she expresses it, she has neglected to follow directions. One such negligence a year is sufficient to give the normal woman a family of ten or twelve children during a lifetime.

While the discontinuance of certain methods is often advised and better ones chosen in their stead, all such advice should be given with the utmost caution and followed only after the most careful consideration.

One general rule stands out above all others. If you have found a method of birth control which is successful and produces no ill effects upon your health or that of your husband, do not change your method. Keep it until you find some adequate reason to change.

Another fact that every woman should remember: The methods advised for birth control are not methods of abortion. When a woman goes to a doctor or a druggist and asks "how to bring herself around," or how to bring about the delayed menstrual period, she is actually asking for something that will bring about an abortion. Often it is innocently assumed that no harm is done if the delay of the monthly period is only one of a few weeks.

I wish to save women the injury done to their health by stating here that drugs and medicines are almost always injurious, and moreover usually fail to produce the results desired. Keep away from drugs! Prevention is the solution of this problem. It is far better for married people, married women especially, to protect themselves from ill-timed and un-desired pregnancy than to indulge in question-able methods of abortion.

One of the most disastrous consequences of a lack of scientific knowledge of birth control is that method used by a certain class of women which consists in "keeping away" from the husband. By this I mean a constant denial of sex communion, inspired by the overwhelming fear of pregnancy. This practice usually brings about the most disastrous consequences. For its evils do not consist merely in the denial of physical intercourse. The poor distracted, worried and hounded wife dares not permit her husband even the ordinary affectionate expres-sion his heart longs for and which his whole body and soul desires and needs. The wife, harried and panic-stricken, dares not even give him a welcoming smile: she shudders at his touch. She struggles against her deepest im-pulses, and meets his tender embrace with a frigid resistance. She dreads the homecoming of her husband, for his presence means not peace but eternal conflict in her heart. I know of one such case, in which both husband and wife agreed to such a policy of married abstinence. Unable to bear the situation the husband, in desperation, went away to war and was killed in the trenches. In the case of another young couple, who lived in the utmost intimacy yet because of their uncertain financial condition did not desire children, the husband, was finally driven to accept a post overseas. After his departure the young wife sank into a condition verging on insanity and had to be sent to a private sanitarium.

There is only one period in the month when these unhappy women have any peace. That is during the menstrual period during which the wife is protected by custom and tradition against the sexual advances of her husband.

If the husband understands and sympathizes with the emotional and nervous strain his loved one is undergoing, he will straightway make it his duty to obtain safe and reliable birth control information and do everything in his power to protect her from this unwholesome fear and worry. It is his duty in any case to find the physician who can diagnose and advise suitable methods.

If, however, the husband is lacking in understanding and is thoughtful only of his own urgent needs, he may meet her resistance by unkind comment, even by brutal retorts and insinuations. He may threaten her by infidelity, and even look elsewhere for a woman to satisfy his passion. It often happens that such men unintentionally fall victims to professional or occasional prostitutes.

Women should not fail to recognize that the sex urge is strong in the male. Sometimes it is as strong, from the biological point of view as the hunger for food. In some men it cannot be controlled by the usual code of morals or the religious and ethical teaching instilled by early training and tradition. Consciously or unconsciously everything is brushed aside by such men in their overwhelming expression of passion. Such men are the slaves of desire instead of its master. Yet such men exist and they are too numerous to count. When their sex urge is not thwarted this savagery in their natures does not reveal itself. The same man may be considered the best of citizens and of parents, as indeed he may in truth be in most respects; but let anything stand in the way of his sexual demands and an entirely unexpected set of characteristics will suddenly be revealed and take possession of him.

Our aim here is not to criticize human nature

but to understand it. Such men reveal a characteristic common to all of us, but under greater control and direction. It is necessary for women to recognize these latent primitive instincts and to recognize their powers even in the best of husbands.

It may not be that the disappointed man will deliberately seek out another woman. But when the sex instinct is stimulated without being satisfied, he is rendered infinitely more susceptible to the attractions of other women. The consequence of such temptations are almost inevitable.

The farseeing wife must be doubly tender to such a husband, proud of the deep primitive energies that are hidden in his nature. Passion is a thing to be proud of. Her problem is to dominate and perhaps sublimate these deep, savage instincts which permeate his being instead of seeking to thwart and deny them. The woman who is wise will seek to find means whereby she can lift his love to the plane of her own where soul communion is desired. His wild passions will thus be directed toward real love and converted into a dynamic instead of destructive creation of happiness in marriage.

CHAPTER XV
THE HUSBAND AS LOVER

There exist a few specially-chosen people who have been endowed with the power and ability of wishing a thing, desiring a thing, willing a thing, so persistently and inexorably that, at last, it has to happen.

—HENRIK IBSEN.

CHAPTER XV

THE HUSBAND AS LOVER

HAPPINESS in marriage must be endlessly recaptured and renewed. It cannot be gained once and held forever in the possession of the husband. Therefore to husbands of all ages—young, middle-aged and even old —these directions are indispensable:

Keep on wooing.

Make the love you have found and which means so much to both of you *your religion.* For it can be the noblest of religions.

Keep your wife eternally youthful. This may seem an impossible task, but it is not and will more than repay you. Happiness is essential for the health and growth of love. Love must keep on growing. It cannot stand still. It grows or it dies. Love cannot thrive in silence. Therefore assure her, reassure her of your deep and growing affection. Good tidings invigorate the flagging energies of a band of explorers; a deep joy enables men and women to transcend the frailties of human weakness. Disappointment, sorrow, depress and disturb the vital functions. Therefore, husband and wife as well, *tell your love* at all times to each other.

Some men do this only occasionally, or when desire is at high tide. They make a grave mistake. Acts may express this love more eloquently than words. But do not, on this account, conclude that words are not necessary also. They are. Love needs constant reassurance. Your wife is in all probability not a mind reader. Unless you tell her, break through the reticence and embarrassment of expressing your thoughts, she may never know what you are thinking and feeling.

This is a greater problem among men who are naturally taciturn and silent, among men who are born and brought up in a tradition which encourages a suppression of stirred emotions. But do not make the mistake of supposing that women do not like to be told over and over again of the love she inspires. This is a story women never tire of hearing. This is a thought all husbands should keep constantly in mind. This is the tonic that rejuvenates and keeps both young.

But, as I have said, words of endearment are

necessary but are not enough. They should not be used to mask neglect in acts.

Support these words of love by careful attention to all the small things concerning the well-being of your beloved.

Does she appear especially pretty to you today? Tell her so.

Has she tried to do some out-of-the-way thing to please you, or to show that she has never forgotten your whims or wishes? Do not fail to let her know that you have noticed this act and that you appreciate the loving thought which has prompted her. This may be something of the most trifling importance. But your failure to recognize the love that has inspired it may cause her the deepest disappointment and subsequent indifference or unhappiness. It may be merely the mending of your clothes, the preparation of your favorite dish, or keeping the baby quiet while you are at rest, or some little economy to save you an added expense. These may be trifles, but they are tremendous trifles, and upon them often depend a woman's happiness and the whole foundation of a happy marriage.

These things may seem small in themselves. But by letting your wife know of your appreciation, you are often removing the burden and the monotony of uninteresting tasks from her mind. Duties that might otherwise be deadly dull are thus transformed by recognition into real pleasures and thus the husband may double the returns of his own love.

Remember that women tire more easily than men. Do everything in your power to spare her strength. Neglect in these matters arouses a natural resentment, and this is bound to rankle. Therefore, when you are about the house, you should indicate by your behavior that you are interested in saving the strength and energy of your wife.

Lifting, reaching, carrying, acts which may seem simple and unimportant to you may have become for your wife through continual routine a burden and a drudgery. In these matters as in all others, thoughtlessness and selfishness through neglect are more costly than the slight trouble prompted by generosity and love. In this respect, I believe that the American husband is the finest in the world, particularly the younger generation of men. Companionship has been attained without any loss of chivalry.

In homes where there are no servants, the household duties such as washing and clearing away the dishes are often shared equally, and the slight burdens become an easily and pleasurably accomplished task.

What were formerly considered exclusively feminine duties seem today to be voluntarily taken on by the husband. Surely there is no loss in manliness or dignity in sharing the heavier and more disagreeable household tasks. In my estimation this mutual acceptance of household duties by the husband as well as the wife does more than any other single thing toward the creation of that splendid comradeship and companionship which are the solidest foundations of permanent homes and happy marriages.

The husband who balks at such tasks and looks upon such duties as essentially feminine, who considers himself henpecked when asked to help in them, is indeed a pathetic creature. He is, moreover, exhibiting an ungenerous and thoughtless side of his nature which will be apprehensively watched by his wife. He cannot know the real joys of true companionship in his married life, and he has himself only to blame when his own action brings out similar traits in his wife. This has been the traditional and unfortunate attitude of many foreign born men toward their wives. Women were not made merely to serve the physical and sexual needs of husbands, with no obligation on the part of the latter except to provide a house and to pay the bills. Fortunately for all of us this type of husband is fast becoming a thing of the past. Small wonder that during the dominance of this type, wives notoriously lost their youth and beauty at a comparatively early age, while today women remain young much longer. This brings me to the point of how much depends upon the love of the husband in the wife's keeping young.

Keep in mind the fact that a woman's heart is ever younger than a man's. The desire to be young and to retain her youth is part of the feminine nature of a woman. There is, scientists tell us, a physiological reverberation in joyous love. To feel that she is loved, that her husband desires her and wants to make her happy will inevitably be reflected in the appearance of your wife.

Your skill as a lover and as a husband is reflected in your wife's appearance. The woman who appears radiant, youthful, glowing with vitality, contentment, and good nature, reveals more of her husband's success than the envious or unhappy wife who may be dressed in the latest fashion or laden with costly jewels, even though this may advertise his financial success. The wife's love-life is reflected in her appearance, her whole attitude toward life. Worry, sleepless, unsatisfied nights, disappointment, all affect her glandular and nervous system, a full and satisfactory love-life making for rejuvenation, a disappointed or thwarted emotional life cruelly writing in her figure and on her face the tragedy of the unhappy and unsatisfied wife. Worry, anxiety, fear, resignation, suspicion, disappointment and concealed hatred age women much more than the mere passing of years. Let all husbands think long over these facts and ponder well their responsibility for them.

Do not forget that your wife desires to be young for your sake. Her desire to be beautiful is to find favor in your eyes. It is but another expression of her love for you. Respond to this love. Help her to keep that attractive and charming quality, if she has it. If by chance she has grown weary of the monotonous routine of petty household or family details and has allowed that quality of attractiveness to slumber, make it your business to *arouse it again to life.*

Even at the expense of sacrifice of other things planned for, encourage her occasionally to buy new and pretty clothes. Most people are too prone to underestimate the spiritual value of such things and yet they ever add a new zest and youth to a woman's life. It is imperative always for a husband to make his wife feel that he is proud to be seen in her company, proud of her looks, of her charm, her style, her dancing, of her cleverness, her wit, her ability, of whatever outstanding quality she possesses and which rendered her so attractive during the days of courtship.

This point cannot be too strongly emphasized. Above all other things, keep alive the *bride* in your wife. Reawaken her ardor, her desire, her love of life. This is the essential and unfailing duty of every husband who must remain first, last, and always the lover.

In the courtship days you sought to find out what gifts, what pleasures, what activities would give the girl you loved most pleasure. Keep this up! To your surprise you may discover that gifts which were pleasing during the

earlier period do not now bring the same spon-
taneous smile of joy.   Why?

A little investigation may reveal to you that
due to self-sacrifice or little hidden econo-
mies, your wife may now be in actual need of
some bit of feminine attire that you know
nothing about.   The bunch of violets that
brought the pink to her cheeks during the days
of courtship may cause only faint or pretended
delight now.   Why is this?   It may be that
before marriage those violets were a symbol to
her of your love, reassuring her of her power
to please you, while now they stab her consciousness into the realization that her whole
wardrobe is shabby or that there is no special
function at which to wear them.   Secretly she
knows of better uses for the money spent, and,
try as she may, she cannot summon to her lips
the same glad smile of courtship days, though
she may not wish to offend you by telling you
of her actual needs.

I know one charming young man, with poetic and romantic longings, but absolutely irre-
sponsible toward the prosaic matters as rent
bills, grocery bills, gas bills and such unpleasant obligations.   Constantly hoping to please
his young wife, he spent money on orchids,

violets, and trinkets of all kinds. These are gestures not to be condemned in themselves; yet in this particular case they did not make the wife happy. Finally she told him that the children needed shoes and that the grocery bills must be paid regularly. The poetic husband sulked. He stopped buying flowers but did not begin to pay the household bills. He had failed to realize that to love fully a woman must be freed from petty worries. Gifts and luxuries are indeed lovely means of accentuating one's love. But the essential requirements of life are also imperative.

It is therefore essential:

1. To establish a household account or budget, so that the wife may know exactly what she can spend to avoid endless worry and anxiety over petty details which may nevertheless become an endless source of bickering and marital discord.

2. To establish an adequate allowance for the wife's personal needs (this in the case where she is not an actual wage-earner).

The regularization of such financial details may be settled once for all time and will automatically remove what might otherwise become an endless source of quarrels and bickerings and may cause profound unhappiness, even disaster.

Large sums of money are often spent for doctors, drugs, medicines or tonics to cure maladies and ailments to the bodies. Marriage is likewise subject to petty ailments and illness which may be cured by the expenditure of trifling sums. Often when the flame of love ebbs low, a temporary separation may be wisely prescribed. Let the wife make a visit occasionally to a friend or family. In other cases, where habit and routine and monotony seem to be on the point of mastering the situation and throttling love once and for all, it would be the safest economy to fling everything aside, to indulge together, lover and beloved, in what might to the unobservant outsider appear as wild extravagance. Sometimes this might consist merely in "stepping out" together, to disappear for a night or a weekend in a spirit of adventure to a new city, attend the theatre, a concert, musical, anything to serve as an antidote to too much tame domesticity. A cure of this character indulged in before the marital discord develops into a storm, may often accomplish miracles in the recapture of marital happiness.